ANTI-INFLAMMATORY RECIPES 2022

QUICK RECIPES TO DECREASE INFLAMMATION

LARA PERRY

Table of Contents

6

Lemon Buttery Shrimp Rice _Servings: 3_

Cooking Time: 10 Minutes

Ingredients:

¼ cup cooked wild rice

½ tsp. Butter divided

¼ tsp. olive oil

1 cup raw shrimps, shelled, deveined, drained ¼ cup frozen peas, thawed, rinsed, drained

1 Tbsp. lemon juice, freshly squeezed

1 Tbsp. chives, minced

Pinch of sea salt, to taste

Directions:

1. Pour ¼ tsp. Butter and oil into wok set over medium heat. Add in shrimps and peas. Sauté until shrimps are coral pink, about 5 to 7

minutes.

2. Add in wild rice and cook until well heated—season with salt and butter.

3. Transfer to a plate. Sprinkle chives and lemon juice on top.

Serve.

Nutrition Info: Calories 510 Carbs: 0g Fat: 0g Protein: 0g

Shrimp-lime Bake With Zucchini And Corn

Servings: 4

Cooking Time: 20 Minutes

Ingredients:

1 tablespoon extra-virgin olive oil

2 small zucchinis, cut into ¼-inch dice

1 cup frozen corn kernels

2 scallions, thinly sliced

1 teaspoon salt

½ teaspoon ground cumin

½ teaspoon chipotle chili powder

1-pound peeled shrimp, thawed if necessary

1 tablespoon finely chopped fresh cilantro

Zest and juice of 1 lime

Directions:

1. Preheat the oven to 400°F. Grease the baking sheet with the oil.

2. On the baking sheet, combine the zucchini, corn, scallions, salt, cumin, and chile powder and mix well. Arrange in a single layer.

3. Add the shrimp on top. Roast within 15 to 20 minutes.

4. Put the cilantro and lime zest and juice, stir to combine, and serve.

Nutrition Info: Calories 184 Total Fat: 5g Total Carbohydrates: 11g Sugar: 3g Fiber: 2g Protein: 26g Sodium: 846mg

Cauliflower Soup _Servings: 10_

Cooking Time: 10 Minutes

Ingredients:

¾ cup of water

2 teaspoon of olive oil

1 onion, diced

1 head of cauliflower, only the florets

1 can of full-fat coconut milk

1 teaspoon of turmeric

1 teaspoon of ginger

1 teaspoon raw honey

Directions:

1. Put all of the fixings into a large stockpot, and boil for about 10

minutes.

2. Use an immersion blender to blend and make the soup smooth.

Serve.

Nutrition Info: Total Carbohydrates 7g Dietary Fiber: 2g Net Carbs: Protein: 2g Total Fat: 11g Calories: 129

Sweet Potato Black Bean Burgers _Servings: 6_

Cooking Time: 10 Minutes

Ingredients:

1/2 jalapeno, seeded and diced

1/2 cup quinoa

6 whole-grain hamburger buns

1 can black beans, rinsed and drained

Olive oil/coconut oil, for cooking

1 sweet potato

1/2 cup red onion, diced

4 tablespoons gluten-free oat flour

2 cloves garlic, minced

2 teaspoons spicy cajun seasoning

1/2 cup cilantro, chopped

1 teaspoon cumin

Sprouts

Salt, to taste

Pepper, to taste

For the Crema:

2 tablespoons cilantro, chopped

1/2 ripe avocado, diced

4 tablespoons low-fat sour cream/plain Greek yogurt 1 teaspoon lime juice

Directions:

1. Rinse quinoa under cold running water. Put a cup of water in a saucepan and heat it. Add quinoa and bring to a boil.

2. Cover, then simmer over low heat until all of the water has absorbed, for about 15 minutes.

3. Turn the heat off and fluff quinoa with a fork. Then transfer quinoa to a bowl and let it cool for 5-10 minutes.

4. Poke potato with a fork and then microwave for a few minutes, until thoroughly cooked and soft. Once cooked, peel the potato and let it cool.

5. Add cooked potato to a food processor along with 1 can black beans, ½ cup chopped cilantro, 2 teaspoons of Cajun seasoning, ½

cup diced onion, 1 teaspoon cumin, and 2 minced cloves of garlic.

Pulse until you obtain a smooth mixture. Transfer it to a bowl and add cooked quinoa.

6. Add in oat flour/oat bran. Mix well and shape into 6 patties. Put patties on a baking sheet and refrigerate for about half an hour.

7. Add all the Crema ingredients to a food processor. Pulse until smooth. Adjust salt to taste and refrigerate.

8. Grease a cooking pan with oil and heat it over medium heat.

Cook each side of patties until light golden, just for 3-4 minutes.

Serve with crema, sprouts, buns, and along with any of your favorite toppings.

Nutrition Info: 206 calories 6 g fat 33.9 g total carbs 7.9 g protein

Coconut Mushroom Soup *Servings: 3*

Cooking Time: 10 Minutes

Ingredients:

1 tablespoon of coconut oil

1 tablespoon of ground ginger

1 cup of cremini mushrooms, chopped

½ teaspoon of turmeric

2 and ½ cups of water

½ cup of canned coconut milk

Sea salt to taste

Directions:

1. Heat-up the coconut oil over medium heat in a large pot, and add the mushrooms. Cook for 3-4 minutes.

2. Put the remaining fixings and boil. Let it simmer for 5 minutes.

3. Divide between three soup bowls, and enjoy!

<u>Nutrition Info:</u> Total Carbohydrates 4g Dietary Fiber: 1g Protein: 2g Total Fat: 14g Calories: 143

Winter Style Fruit Salad _Servings: 6_

Cooking Time: 0 Minutes

Ingredients:

4 cooked sweet potatoes, cubed (1-inch cubes) 3 pears, cubed (1-inch cubes)

1 cup of grapes, halved

1 apple, cubed

½ cup of pecan halves

2 tablespoons of olive oil

1 tablespoon of red wine vinegar

2 tablespoons of raw honey

Directions:

1. Mix the olive oil, red wine vinegar, then the raw honey to make the dressing, and set aside.

2. Combine the chopped fruit, sweet potato, and pecan halves, and divide this between six serving bowls. Drizzle each bowl with the dressing.

<u>Nutrition Info:</u> Total Carbohydrates 40g Dietary Fiber: 6g Protein: 3g Total Fat: 11g Calories: 251

Honey-roasted Chicken Thighs With Carrots

Servings: 4

Cooking Time: 50 Minutes

Ingredients:

2 tablespoons unsalted butter, at room temperature 3 large carrots, thinly sliced

2 garlic cloves, minced

4 bone-in, skin-on chicken thighs

1 teaspoon salt

½ teaspoon dried rosemary

¼ teaspoon freshly ground black pepper

2 tablespoons honey

1 cup chicken broth or vegetable broth

Lemon wedges, for serving

Directions:

1. Preheat the oven to 400°F. Grease the baking sheet with the butter.

2. Arrange the carrots and garlic in a single layer on the baking sheet.

3. Put the chicken, skin-side up, on top of the vegetables, and season with the salt, rosemary, and pepper.

4. Put the honey on top and add the broth.

5. Roast within 40 to 45 minutes. Remove, then let it rest for 5

minutes, and serve with lemon wedges.

Nutrition Info: Calories 428 Total Fat: 28g Total Carbohydrates: 15g Sugar: 11g Fiber: 2g Protein: 30g Sodium: 732mg

Turkey Chili _Servings: 8_

Cooking Time: 4 Hours And 10 Minutes

Ingredients:

1-pound ground turkey, preferably 99% lean

2 cans of red kidney beans, rinsed & drained (15 oz each) 1 red pepper, chopped

2 cans of tomato sauce (15 oz each)

1 jar deli-sliced tamed jalapeno peppers, drained (16 oz) 2 cans of petite tomatoes, diced (15 oz each) 1 tablespoon cumin

1 yellow pepper, roughly chopped

2 cans of black beans, preferably rinsed & drained (15 oz each) 1 cup corn, frozen

2 tablespoon chili powder

1 tablespoon olive oil

Black pepper & salt to taste

1 medium onion, diced

Green onions, avocado, shredded cheese, Greek yogurt/sour cream, to top, optional

Directions:

1. Warm the oil until hot in a large skillet. Once done, carefully place the turkey into the hot skillet & cook until turn brown. Pour the turkey into the bottom of your slow cooker, preferably 6 quarts.

2. Add the jalapeños, corn, peppers, onion, diced tomatoes, tomato sauce, beans, cumin, and chili powder. Mix, then put pepper and salt to taste.

3. Cover & cook for 6 hours on low heat or 4 hours on high heat.

Serve with the optional toppings and enjoy.

Nutrition Info: kcal 455 Fat: 9 g Fiber: 19 g Protein: 38 g

Lentil Soup With Spices *Servings: 5*

Cooking Time: 25 Minutes

Ingredients:

1 Cup of yellow onion (cut into cubes)

1 Cup of carrot (cut into cubes)

1 Cup of turnip

2tbsp extra-virgin olive oil

2tbsp balsamic vinegar

4 cups of baby spinach

2 cups brown lentils

¼ Cup of fresh parsley

Directions:

1. Preheat the pressure cooker on medium flame and add olive oil and vegetables in it.

2. After 5 minutes, add broth, lentils, and salt in the pot and simmer for 15 minutes.

3. Remove the lid and add spinach and vinegar in it.

4. Stir the soup for 5 minutes and turn off the flame.

5. Garnish it with fresh parsley.

Nutrition Info: Calories 96 Carbs: 16g Fat: 1g Protein: 4g

Garlicky Chicken And Vegetables _Servings: 4_

Cooking Time: 45 Minutes

Ingredients:

2 teaspoons extra-virgin olive oil

1 leek, white part only, thinly sliced

2 large zucchinis, cut into ¼-inch slices

4 bone-in, skin-on chicken breasts

3 garlic cloves, minced

1 teaspoon salt

1 teaspoon dried oregano

¼ teaspoon freshly ground black pepper

½ cup white wine

Juice of 1 lemon

Directions:

1. Preheat the oven to 400°F. Grease the baking sheet with the oil.

2. Place the leek and zucchini on the baking sheet.

3. Put the chicken, skin-side up, and sprinkle with the garlic, salt, oregano, and pepper. Add the wine.

4. Roast within 35 to 40 minutes. Remove and let rest for 5 minutes.

5. Add the lemon juice and serve.

Nutrition Info: Calories 315 Total Fat: 8g Total Carbohydrates: 12g Sugar: 4g Fiber: 2g Protein: 44g Sodium: 685mg

Smoked Salmon Salad _Servings: 4_

Cooking Time: 20 Minutes

Ingredients:

2 baby fennel bulbs, thinly sliced, some fronds reserved 1 tablespoon salted baby capers, rinsed, drained ½ cup natural yogurt

2 tablespoons parsley, chopped

1 tablespoon lemon juice, freshly squeezed

2 tablespoons fresh chives, chopped

1 tablespoon chopped fresh tarragon

180g sliced smoked salmon, low-salt

½ red onion, sliced thinly

1 teaspoon lemon rind, finely grated

½ cup French green lentils, rinsed

60g fresh baby spinach

½ avocado, sliced

A pinch of caster sugar

Directions:

1. Put water in a large saucepan with water and boil over moderate heat. Once boiling; cook the lentils until tender, for 20 minutes; drain well.

2. In the meantime, heat a chargrill pan over high heat in advance.

Spray the fennel slices with some oil & cook until tender, for 2

minutes per side.

3. Process the chives, parsley, yogurt, tarragon, lemon rind, and capers in a food processor until completely smooth and then season with pepper to taste.

4. Place the onion with sugar, juice & a pinch of salt in a large-sized mixing bowl. Set aside for a couple of minutes and then drain.

5. Combine the lentils with onion, fennel, avocado, and spinach in a large-sized mixing bowl. Evenly divide among the plates and then top with the fish. Sprinkle with the leftover fennel fronds & more of fresh parsley. Drizzle with the green goddess dressing. Enjoy.

Nutrition Info: kcal 368 Fat: 14 g Fiber: 8 g Protein: 20 g

Bean Shawarma Salad _Servings: 2_

Cooking Time: 20 Minutes

Ingredients:

For Preparing Salad

20 Pita chips

5-ounces Spring lettuce

10 Cherry tomatoes

¾ Cup fresh parsley

¼ Cup red onion (chop)

For Chickpeas

1tbsp Olive oil

1 Heading-tbsp cumin and turmeric

½ Heading-tbsp paprika and coriander powder 1 Pinch black pepper

½ Scant Kosher salt

¼tbsp Ginger and cinnamon powder

For Preparing Dressing

3 Garlic Cloves

1tbsp Dried drill

1tbsp Lime juice

Water

½ Cup hummus

Directions:

1. Place a rack in the already preheated oven (204C). Mix chickpeas with all spices and herbs.

2. Place a thin layer of chickpeas on the baking sheet and bake it almost for 20 minutes. Bake it until the beans are golden brown.

3. For preparing the dressing, mix all ingredients in a whisking bowl and blend it. Add water gradually for appropriate smoothness.

4. Mix all herbs and spices for preparing salad.

5. For serving, add pita chips and beans in the salad and drizzle some dressing over it.

Nutrition Info: Calories 173 Carbs: 8g Fat: 6g Protein: 19g

Pineapple Fried Rice _Servings: 4_

Cooking Time: 20 Minutes

Ingredients:

2 carrots, peeled and grated

2 green onions, sliced

3 tablespoons soy sauce

1/2 cup ham, diced

1 tablespoon sesame oil

2 cups canned/fresh pineapple, diced

1/2 teaspoon ginger powder

3 cups brown rice, cooked

1/4 teaspoon white pepper

2 tablespoons olive oil

1/2 cup frozen peas

2 garlic cloves, minced

1/2 cup frozen corn

1 onion, diced

Directions:

1. Put 1 tablespoon sesame oil, 3 tablespoons soy sauce, 2 pinches of white pepper, and 1/2 teaspoon ginger powder in a bowl. Mix well and keep it aside.

2. Preheat oil in a skillet. Add the garlic along with the diced onion.

Cook for about 3-4 minutes, stirring often.

3. Add 1/2 cup frozen peas, grated carrots, and 1/2 cup frozen corn.

Stir until veggies are tender, just for few minutes.

4. Stir in soy sauce mixture, 2 cups of diced pineapple, ½ cup chopped ham, 3 cups cooked brown rice, and sliced green onions.

Cook for about 2-3 minutes, stirring often. Serve!

Nutrition Info: 252 calories 12.8 g fat 33 g total carbs 3 g protein

Lentil Soup Servings: 2

Cooking Time: 30 Minutes

Ingredients:

2 Carrots, medium & diced

2 tbsp. Lemon Juice, fresh

1 tbsp. Turmeric Powder

1/3 cup Lentils, cooked

1 tbsp. Almonds, chopped

1 Celery Stalk, diced

1 bunch of Parsley, chopped freshly

1 Yellow Onion, large & chopped

Black Pepper, freshly grounded

1 Parsnip, medium & chopped

½ tsp. Cumin Powder

3 ½ cups Water

½ tsp. Pink Himalayan Salt

4 kale leaves, chopped roughly

Directions:

1. To start with, place carrots, parsnip, one tablespoon of water and onion in a medium-sized pot over medium heat.

2. Cook the vegetable mixture for 5 minutes while stirring it occasionally.

3. Next, stir in the lentils and spices into it. Combine well.

4. After that, pour water to the pot and bring the mixture to a boil.

5. Now, reduce the heat to low and allow it to simmer for 20

minutes.

6. Off the heat and remove it from the stove. Add the kale, lemon juice, parsley, and salt to it.

7. Then, give a good stir until everything comes together.

8. Top it with almonds and serve it hot.

Nutrition Info: Calories: 242KcalProteins: 10gCarbohydrates: 46gFat: 4g

Delicious Tuna Salad <u>Servings: 2</u>

Cooking Time: 15 Minutes

Ingredients:

2 cans tuna packed in water (5oz each), drained ¼ cup mayonnaise

2 tablespoons fresh basil, chopped

1 tablespoon lemon juice, freshly squeezed

2 tablespoons fire-roasted red peppers, chopped ¼ cup kalamata or mixed olives, chopped

2 large vine-ripened tomatoes

1 tablespoon capers

2 tablespoons red onion, minced

Pepper & salt to taste

Directions:

1. Add all the items (except tomatoes) together in a large-sized mixing bowl; give the ingredients a good stir until combined well.

Slice the tomatoes into sixths and then gently pry it open. Scoop the prepared tuna salad mixture into the middle; serve immediately & enjoy.

<u>Nutrition Info:</u> kcal 405 Fat: 24 g Fiber: 3.2 g Protein: 37 g

Aioli With Eggs _Servings: 12_

Cooking Time: 0 Minutes

Ingredients:

2 egg yolks

1 garlic, grated

2 Tbsp. water

½ cup extra virgin olive oil

¼ cup lemon juice, fresh squeezed, pips removed ¼ tsp. sea salt

Dash of cayenne pepper powder

Pinch of white pepper, to taste

Directions:

1. Pour garlic, egg yolks, salt, and water into blender; process until smooth. Put in olive oil in a slow stream until dressing emulsifies.

2. Add in remaining ingredients. Taste; adjust seasoning if needed.

Pour into an airtight container; use as needed.

Nutrition Info: Calories 100 Carbs: 1g Fat: 11g Protein: 0g

Spaghetti Pasta With Herbed Mushroom Sauce

Ingredients:

200 grams/6.3 oz around a large portion of a pack of wheat slender spaghetti *

140 grams cleaned cleaved mushrooms 12-15 pieces*

¼ cup cream

3 cups milk

2 tablespoon cooking olive oil in addition to 2 teaspoon more oil or liquefied margarine to include mid-way 1.5 tablespoon flour

½ cup cleaved onions

¼ to ½ cup crisply ground parmesan cheddar

Couple of bits of dark pepper

Salt to taste

2 teaspoons dried or new thyme *

Bunch of chiffonade new basil leaves

Directions:

1. Cook pasta still somewhat firm as indicated by the bundle.

2. While the pasta is cooking, we should begin making the sauce.

3. Warmth the 3 cups milk in the microwave for 3 minutes or on the stovetop until a stew.

4. At the same time heat 2 tablespoon oil in a non-stick container on medium high and cook the cleaved mushrooms. Cook for around 2

minutes.

5. From the outset the mushrooms will discharge some water, then it will evaporate in the long run and become fresh apiece.

6. Presently lessen the fire to medium include the onions and cook for 1 moment.

7. Presently include 2 teaspoons of softened spread and sprinkle some flour.

8. Mix for 20 seconds.

9. Include the warm milk mixing constantly to shape a smooth sauce.

10. When the sauce thicken i.e. goes to a stew, switch off the fire.

11. Presently include ¼ cup ground parmesan cheddar. Mix until smooth. For 30 seconds.

12. Presently include the salt, pepper and thyme.

13. Give a trial. Modify flavoring if necessary.

14. In interim pasta ought to be bubbled still somewhat firm.

15. Strain the warm water in a colander. Keep the tap running and pour cold water to stop it's cooking, channel all the water and hurl it with the sauce.

16. If not eating promptly, don't blend the pasta in the sauce. Keep the pasta separate, covered with oil and secured.

17. Serve warm with more sprinkle of parmesan cheddar.

Appreciate!

Brown Rice And Shitake Miso Soup With Scallions

Servings: 4

Cooking Time: 45 Minutes

Ingredients:

2 tablespoons sesame oil

1 cup thinly sliced shiitake mushroom caps

1 garlic clove, minced

1 (1½-inch) piece fresh ginger, peeled and sliced 1 cup medium-grain brown rice

½ teaspoon salt

1 tablespoon white miso

2 scallions, thinly sliced

2 tablespoons finely chopped fresh cilantro <u>Directions:</u>

1. Heat-up the oil over medium-high heat in a large pot.

2. Add the mushrooms, garlic, and ginger and sauté until the mushrooms begin to soften about 5 minutes.

3. Put the rice and stir to coat with the oil evenly. Add 2 cups of water and salt and boil.

4. Simmer within 30 to 40 minutes. Use a little of the soup broth to soften the miso, then stir it into the pot until well blended.

5. Mix in the scallions plus cilantro, then serve.

Nutrition Info: Calories 265 Total Fat: 8g Total Carbohydrates: 43g Sugar: 2g Fiber: 3g Protein: 5g Sodium: 456mg

Barbecued Ocean Trout With Garlic And Parsley Dressing

Servings: 8

Cooking Time: 25 Minutes

Ingredients:

3 ½ pounds piece of trout fillet, preferably ocean trout, boned, skin on

4 cloves of garlic, sliced thinly

2 tablespoons capers, coarsely chopped

½ cup flat-leaf parsley leaves, fresh

1 red chili, preferably long; sliced thinly 2 tablespoons lemon juice, freshly squeezed ½ cup olive oil

Lemon wedges, to serve

Directions:

1. Brush the trout with approximately 2 tablespoons of oil; ensure that all sides are coated nicely. Preheat your barbecue over high heat, preferably with a closed hood. Decrease the heat to medium; place the coated trout on the barbecue plate, preferably on the skin-side. Cook until partially cooked

and turn golden, for a couple of minutes. Carefully turn the trout; cook until cooked through, for 12 to 15 minutes, with the hood closed. Transfer the fillet to a large-sized serving platter.

2. In the meantime, heat the leftover oil; garlic over low heat in a small-sized saucepan until just heated through; garlic begins to change its color. Remove, then stir in the capers, lemon juice, chili.

Drizzle the trout with the prepared dressing and then sprinkle with the fresh parsley leaves. Immediately serve with fresh lemon wedges, enjoy.

Nutrition Info: kcal 170 Fat: 30 g Fiber: 2 g Protein: 37 g

Curried Cauliflower And Chickpea Wraps

Ingredients:

1 Ginger Fresh

2 cloves Garlic

1 can Chickpeas

1 Red Onion

8 ounces Cauliflower Florets

1 teaspoon Garam Masala

2 tablespoons Arrowroot Starch

1 Lemon

1 pack Cilantro Fresh

1/4 cup Vegan Yogurt

4 Wraps

3 tablespoons Shredded Coconut

4 ounces Baby Spinach

1 tablespoon Vegetable Oil

1 teaspoon Salt and Pepper To taste

Directions:

1. Preheat the stove to 400 °F (205 °C). Strip and mince 1 tsp of the ginger. Mince the garlic. Channel and wash the chickpeas. Strip and meagerly cut the red onion. Split the lemon.

2. Coat a heating sheet with 1 tbsp vegetable oil. In an enormous bowl, consolidate the minced ginger, garlic, the juice from a large portion of the lemon, chickpeas, cut red onion, cauliflower florets, garam masala, arrowroot starch, and 1/2 tsp salt. Move to the preparing sheet and meal in the broiler until cauliflower is delicate and sautéed in places, around 20 to 25 minutes.

3. Hack the cilantro leaves and delicate stems. In a little bowl, whisk together the cilantro, yogurt, 1 tbsp lemon juice, and a spot of salt and pepper.

4. Spot the encloses by foil and pop them into the stove to warm around 3 to 4 minutes.

5. Spot a little nonstick skillet over medium warmth and include the destroyed coconut. Toast, shaking the dish habitually until daintily cooked, around 2 to 3 minutes.

6. Gap the infant spinach and cooked vegetables between the warm wraps. Lay the cauliflower chickpea wraps on enormous plates and sprinkle with the cilantro sauce.Sprinkle with toasted coconut

Buckwheat Noodle Soup _Servings: 4_

Cooking Time: 25 Minutes

Ingredients:

2 cups Bok Choy, chopped

3 tbsp. Tamari

3 bundles of Buckwheat Noodles

2 cups Edamame Beans

7 oz. Shiitake Mushrooms, chopped

4 cups Water

1 tsp. Ginger, grated

Dash of Salt

1 Garlic Clove, grated

Directions:

1. First, place water, ginger, soy sauce, and garlic in a medium-sized pot over medium heat.

2. Bring the ginger-soy sauce mixture to a boil and then stir in the edamame and shiitake to it.

3. Continue cooking for further 7 minutes or until tender.

4. Next, cook the soba noodles by following the Directions: given in the packet until cooked. Wash and drain well.

5. Now, add the bok choy to shiitake mixture and cook for further one minute or until the bok choy is wilted.

6. Finally, divide the soba noodles among the serving bowls and top it with the mushroom mixture.

Nutrition Info: Calories: 234KcalProteins: 14.2gCarbohydrates: 35.1gFat: 4g

Easy Salmon Salad _Servings: 1_

Cooking Time: 0 Minutes

Ingredients:

1 cup of organic arugula

1 can of wild-caught salmon

½ of an avocado, sliced

1 tablespoon of olive oil

1 teaspoon of Dijon mustard

1 teaspoon of sea salt

Directions:

1. Start by whisking the olive oil, Dijon mustard, and sea salt together in a mixing bowl to make the dressing. Set aside.

2. Assemble the salad with the arugula as the base, and top with the salmon and sliced avocado.

3. Drizzle with the dressing.

Nutrition Info: Total Carbohydrates 7g Dietary Fiber: 5g Protein: 48g Total Fat: 37g Calories: 553

Vegetable Soup <u>Servings: 4</u>

Cooking Time: 40 Minutes

Ingredients:

1 tbsp. Coconut Oil

2 cups Kale, chopped

2 Celery Stalks, diced

½ of 15 oz. can of White Beans, drained & rinsed 1 Onion, large & diced

¼ tsp. Black Pepper

1 Carrot, medium & diced

2 cups Cauliflower, cut into florets

1 tsp. Turmeric, grounded

1 tsp. Sea Salt

3 Garlic cloves, minced

6 cups Vegetable Broth

Directions:

1. To start with, heat oil in a large pot over medium-low heat.

2. Stir in the onion to the pot and sauté it for 5 minutes or until softened.

3. Put the carrot plus celery to the pot and continue cooking for another 4 minutes or until the veggies softened.

4. Now, spoon in the turmeric, garlic, and ginger to the mixture. Stir well.

5. Cook the veggie mixture for 1 minute or until fragrant.

6. Then, pour the vegetable broth along with salt and pepper and bring the mixture to a boil.

7. Once it starts boiling, add the cauliflower. Reduce the heat and simmer the vegetable mixture for 13 to 15 minutes or until the cauliflower is softened.

8. Finally, add the beans and kale—Cook within 2 minutes.

9. Serve it hot.

Nutrition Info: Calories 192Kcal Proteins:12.6g Carbohydrates: 24.6g Fat: 6.4g

Lemony Garlic Shrimp Servings: 4

Cooking Time: 15 Minutes

Ingredients:

1 and ¼ pounds shrimp, boiled or steamed

3 tablespoons garlic, minced

¼ cup lemon juice

2 tablespoons olive oil

¼ cup parsley

Directions:

1. Take a small skillet and place it over medium heat, add garlic and oil and stir cook for 1 minute.

2. Add parsley, lemon juice and season with salt and pepper accordingly.

3. Add shrimp in a large bowl and transfer the mixture from the skillet over the shrimp.

4. Chill and serve.

Nutrition Info: Calories: 130Fat: 3gCarbohydrates: 2gProtein: 22g

Blt Spring Rolls Ingredients:

new lettuce, torn pieces or slashed

avocado cuts, discretionary

SESAME-SOY DIPPING SAUCE

1/4 cup Soy Sauce

1/4 cup cold water

1 Tablespoon Mayonnaise (discretionary, this makes the plunge velvety)

1 teaspoon new Lime Juice

1 teaspoon Sesame Oil

1 teaspoon sriracha sauce or any hot sauce (discretionary) Directions:

1. medium tomato (seeded and cut 1/4" thick) 2. pieces bacon, cooked

3. new basil, mint or different herbs

4. rice paper

Brisket With Blue Cheese _Servings: 6_

Cooking Time: 8 Hrs. 10 Minutes

Ingredients:

1 cup of water

1/2 tbsp garlic paste

1/4 cup soy sauce

1 ½ lb. corned beef brisket

1/3 teaspoon ground coriander

1/4 teaspoon cloves, ground

1 tbsp olive oil

1 shallot, chopped

2 oz. blue cheese, crumbled

Cooking spray

Directions:

1. Place a pan over moderate heat and add oil to heat.

2. Toss in shallots and stir and cook for 5 minutes.

3. Stir in garlic paste and cook for 1 minute.

4. Transfer it to the slow cooker, greased with cooking spray.

5. Place brisket in the same pan and sear until golden from both sides.

6. Transfer the beef to the slow cooker along with other ingredients except for cheese.

7. Put on its lid and cook for 8 hrs. on low heat.

8. Garnish with cheese and serve.

<u>Nutrition Info:</u> Calories 397, Protein 23.5g, Fat 31.4g, Carbs 3.9g, Fiber 0 g

Cold Soba With Miso Dressing_Ingredients:

6oz buckwheat Soba noodles

1/2 cups destroyed carrots

1 cup solidified shelled edamame, defrosted 2 Persian cucumbers, cut

1 cup hacked cilantro

1/4 cup sesame seeds

2 tbsp dark sesame seeds

White Miso Dressing (makes 2 cups)

2/3 cup white miso glue

Juice of 2 medium size lemons

4 tbsp rice vinegar

4 tbsp additional virgin olive oil

4 tbsp squeezed orange

2 tbsp new ground ginger

2 tbsp maple syrup

Directions:

1. Cook soba noodles as per the guidelines in the bundling (make a point not to overcook them or they will get sticky and remain together). Channel well and move to an enormous bowl 2. Include destroyed carrots, edamame, cucumber, cilantro and sesame seeds

3. To set up the dressing, consolidate every one of the fixings in a blender. Mix until smooth

4. Pour wanted measure of dressing over the noodles (we utilized about a cup and a half)

Baked Buffalo Cauliflower Chunks _Servings: 2_

Cooking Time: 35 Minutes

Ingredients:

¼-cup water

¼-cup banana flour

A pinch of salt and pepper

1-pc medium cauliflower, cut into bite-size pieces ½-cup hot sauce

2-Tbsp.s butter, melted

Blue cheese or ranch dressing (optional)

Directions:

1. Preheat your oven to 425°F. Meanwhile, line a baking pan with foil.

2. Combine the water, flour, and a pinch of salt and pepper in a large mixing bowl.

3. Mix well until thoroughly combined.

4. Add the cauliflower; toss to coat thoroughly.

5. Transfer the mixture to the baking pan. Bake for 15 minutes, flipping once.

6. While baking, combine the hot sauce and butter in a small bowl.

7. Pour the sauce over the baked cauliflower.

8. Return the baked cauliflower to the oven, and bake further for 20 minutes.

9. Serve immediately with a ranch dressing on the side, if desired.

Nutrition Info: Calories: 168Cal Fat: 5.6gProtein: 8.4gCarbs: 23.8gFiber: 2.8g

Garlic Chicken Bake With Basil &tomatoes

Servings: 4

Cooking Time: 30 Minutes

Ingredients:

½ medium yellow onion

2tbsp Olive oil

3 Minced Garlic Cloves

1 Cup Basil (loosely cut)

1.lb Boneless chicken breast

14.5-ounces Italian chop tomatoes

Salt & pepper

4 Medium zucchinis (spiralized into noodles) 1tbsp crushed red pepper

2tbsp Olive oil

Directions:

1. Pound the chicken pieces with a pan for fast cooking. Sprinkle salt, pepper, and oil on chicken pieces and marinate both sides of chicken equally.

2. Fry chicken pieces on a large hot skillet for 2-3 minutes on each side.

3. Sautee onion in the same skillet pan until it's brown. Add tomatoes, basil leaves, and garlic in it.

4. Simmer it for 3 minutes and add all spices and chicken in the skillet.

5. Serve it on the plate along with saucy zoodles.

Nutrition Info: Calories 44 Carbs: 7g Fat: 0g Protein: 2g

Creamy Turmeric Cauliflower Soup <u>*Servings: 4*</u>

Cooking Time: 15 Minutes

Ingredients:

2 tablespoons extra-virgin olive oil

1 leek, white part only, thinly sliced

3 cups cauliflower florets

1 garlic clove, peeled

1 (1¼-inch) piece fresh ginger, peeled and sliced 1½ teaspoons turmeric

½ teaspoon salt

¼ teaspoon freshly ground black pepper

¼ teaspoon ground cumin

3 cups vegetable broth

1 cup full-Fat: coconut milk

¼ cup finely chopped fresh cilantro

Directions:

1. Heat-up the oil over high heat in a large pot.

2. Sauté the leek within 3 to 4 minutes.

3. Put the cauliflower, garlic, ginger, turmeric, salt, pepper, and cumin and sauté for 1 to 2 minutes.

4. Put the broth, and boil.

5. Simmer within 5 minutes.

6. Purée the soup using an immersion blender until smooth.

7. Stir in the coconut milk and cilantro, heat through, and serve.

Nutrition Info: Calories 264 Total Fat: 23g Total Carbohydrates: 12g Sugar: 5g Fiber: 4g Protein: 7g Sodium: 900mg

Mushroom, Kale, And Sweet Potato Brown Rice

Servings: 4

Cooking Time: 50 Minutes

Ingredients:

¼ cup extra-virgin olive oil

4 cups coarsely chopped kale leaves

2 leeks, white parts only, thinly sliced

1 cup sliced mushrooms

2 garlic cloves, minced

2 cups peeled sweet potatoes cut into ½-inch dice 1 cup of brown rice

2 cups vegetable broth

1 teaspoon salt

¼ teaspoon freshly ground black pepper

¼ cup freshly squeezed lemon juice

2 tablespoons finely chopped fresh flat-leaf parsley Directions:

1. Heat the oil over high heat.

2. Add the kale, leeks, mushrooms, and garlic and sauté until soft, about 5 minutes.

3. Add the sweet potatoes and rice and sauté for about 3 minutes.

4. Add the broth, salt, and pepper and boil. Simmer within 30 to 40 minutes.

5. Combine in the lemon juice and parsley, then serve.

Nutrition Info: Calories 425 Fat: 15g Total Carbohydrates: 65g Sugar: 6g Fiber: 6g Protein: 11g Sodium: 1045mg

Baked Tilapia Recipe With Pecan Rosemary Topping

Servings: 4

Cooking Time: 20 Minutes

Ingredients:

4 tilapia fillets (4 ounces each)

½ teaspoon brown sugar or coconut palm sugar 2 teaspoons fresh rosemary, chopped

1/3 cup raw pecans, chopped

A pinch of cayenne pepper

1 ½ teaspoon olive oil

1 large egg white

1/8 teaspoon salt

1/3 cup panko breadcrumbs, preferably whole-wheat Directions:

1. Heat-up your oven to 350 F.

2. Stir the pecans with breadcrumbs, coconut palm sugar, rosemary, cayenne pepper, and salt in a small-sized baking dish. Add the olive oil; toss.

3. Bake within 7 to 8 minutes, until the mixture turns light golden brown.

4. Adjust the heat to 400 F and coat a large-sized glass baking dish with some cooking spray.

5. Whisk the egg white in the shallow dish. Work in batches; dip the fish (one tilapia at a time) into the egg white, and then, coating lightly into the pecan mixture. Put the coated fillets in the baking dish.

6. Press the leftover pecan mixture over the tilapia fillets.

7. Bake within 8 to 10 minutes. Serve immediately & enjoy.

Nutrition Info: kcal 222 Fat: 10 g Fiber: 2 g Protein: 27 g

Black Bean Tortilla Wrap _Servings: 2_

Cooking Time: 0 Minutes

Ingredients:

¼ cup of corn

1 handful of fresh basil

½ cup of arugula

1 tablespoon of nutritional yeast

¼ cup of canned black beans

1 peach, sliced

1 teaspoon of lime juice

2 gluten-free tortillas

Directions:

1. Divide the beans, corn, arugula, and peaches between the two tortillas.

2. Top each tortilla with half the fresh basil and lime juice <u>Nutrition Info:</u>
Total Carbohydrates 44g Dietary Fiber: 7g Protein: 8g Total Fat: 1g Calories:
203

White Bean Chicken With Winter Green Vegetables

Servings: 8

Cooking Time: 45 Minutes

Ingredients:

4 Garlic cloves

1tbsp Olive oil

3 medium parsnips

1kg Small cubes of chicken

1 Teaspoon cumin powder

2 Leaks & 1 Green part

2 Carrots (cut into cubes)

1 ¼ White kidney beans (overnight soaked)

½ Teaspoon dried oregano

2 Teaspoon Kosher salt

Cilantro leaves

1 1/2tbsp Ground ancho chilies

Directions:

1. Cook garlic, leeks, chicken, and olive oil in a large pot on a medium flame for 5 minutes.

2. Now add carrots and parsnips, and after stirring for 2 minutes, add all seasoning ingredients.

3. Stir until the fragrant starts coming from it.

4. Now add beans and 5 cups of water in the pot.

5. Bring it to a boil and reduce the flame.

6. Allow it to simmer almost for 30 minutes and garnish with parsley and cilantro leaves.

Nutrition Info: Calories 263 Carbs: 24g Fat: 7g Protein: 26g

Herbed Baked Salmon _Servings: 2_

Cooking Time: 15 Minutes

Ingredients:

10 oz. Salmon Fillet

1 tsp. Olive Oil

1 tsp. Honey

1 tsp. Tarragon, fresh

1/8 tsp. Salt

2 tsp. Dijon Mustard

¼ tsp. Thyme, dried

¼ tsp. Oregano, dried

Directions:

1. Preheat the oven to 425 ˚ F.

2. After that, combine all the ingredients, excluding the salmon in a medium-sized bowl.

3. Now, spoon this mixture evenly over the salmon.

4. Then, place the salmon with the skin side down on the parchment paper-lined baking sheet.

5. Finally, bake for 8 minutes or until the fish flakes.

<u>Nutrition Info:</u> Calories: 239KcalProteins: 31gCarbohydrates: 3gFat: 11g

Greek Yogurt Chicken Salad

Ingredients:

Chopped chicken

Green apple

Red onion

Celery

Dried cranberries

Directions:

1. Greek yogurt chicken serving of mixed greens is such an extraordinary supper prep lunch thought. You can place it in an artisan jostle and eat only that or you can pack it in a super prep compartment with more veggies, chips, and so forth. Here are some serving recommendations.

2. On a bit of toast

3. In a tortilla with lettuce

4. With chips or saltines

5. In a bit of ice burg lettuce (low carb choice!)

Pounded Chickpea Salad

Ingredients:

1 avocado

1/2 crisp lemon

1 can chickpeas depleted (19 oz)

1/4 cup cut red onion

2 cups grape tomatoes cut

2 cups diced cucumber

1/2 cup crisp parsley

3/4 cup diced green chime pepper

Dressing

1/4 cup olive oil

2 tablespoons red wine vinegar

1/2 teaspoon cumin

salt and pepper

Directions:

1. Cut avocado into 3D squares and spot in bowl. Press the juice from 1/2 lemon over the avocado and delicately mix to consolidate.

2. Include remaining serving of mixed greens ingredients and delicately hurl to join.

3. Refrigerate at any rate one hour before serving.

Valencia Salad *Servings: 10*

Cooking Time: 0 Minutes

Ingredients:

1 tsp. Kalamata olives in oil, pitted, drained lightly, halved, julienned

1 head, small Romaine lettuce, rinsed, spun-dried, sliced into bite-sized pieces

½ piece, small shallot, julienned

1 tsp. Dijon mustard

½ small satsuma or tangerine, pulp only

1 tsp. white wine vinegar

1 tsp. extra virgin olive oil

1 pinch fresh thyme, minced

Pinch of sea salt

Pinch of black pepper, to taste

Directions:

1. Combine vinegar, oil, fresh thyme, salt, mustard, black pepper, and honey, if using. Whisk well until dressing emulsifies a little.

2. Toss together the remaining salad ingredients in a salad bowl.

3. Drizzle dressing on top when about to serve. Serve immediately with 1 slice if sugar-free sourdough bread or saltine.

<u>Nutrition Info:</u> Calories 238 Carbs: 23g Fat: 15g Protein: 8g

"Eat Your Greens" Soup _Servings: 4_

Cooking Time: 20 Minutes

Ingredients:

¼ cup extra-virgin olive oil

2 leeks, white parts only, thinly sliced

1 fennel bulb, trimmed and thinly sliced

1 garlic clove, peeled

1 bunch Swiss chard, coarsely chopped

4 cups coarsely chopped kale

4 cups coarsely chopped mustard greens

3 cups vegetable broth

2 tablespoons apple cider vinegar

1 teaspoon salt

¼ teaspoon freshly ground black pepper

¼ cup chopped cashews (optional)

Directions:

1. Heat-up the oil over high heat in a large pot.

2. Add the leeks, fennel, and garlic and sauté until softened, for about 5 minutes.

3. Add the Swiss chard, kale, and mustard greens and sauté until the greens wilt, 2 to 3 minutes.

4. Put the broth and boil.

5. Simmer within 5 minutes.

6. Stir in the vinegar, salt, pepper, and cashews (if using).

7. Purée the soup using an immersion blender until smooth and serve.

Nutrition Info: Calories 238 Total Fat: 14g Total Carbohydrates: 22g Sugar: 4g Fiber: 6g Protein: 9g Sodium: 1294mg

Miso Salmon And Green Beans _Servings: 4_

Cooking Time: 25 Minutes

Ingredients:

1 tablespoon sesame oil

1-pound green beans, trimmed

1-pound skin-on salmon fillets, cut into 4 steaks ¼ cup white miso

2 teaspoons gluten-free tamari or soy sauce 2 scallions, thinly sliced

Directions:

1. Preheat the oven to 400°F. Grease the baking sheet with the oil.

2. Put the green beans, then the salmon on top of the green beans, and brush each piece with the miso.

3. Roast within 20 to 25 minutes.

4. Drizzle with the tamari, sprinkle with the scallions, and serve.

Nutrition Info: Calories 213 Total Fat: 7g Total Carbohydrates: 13g Sugar: 3g Fiber: 5g Protein: 27g Sodium: 989mg

Leek, Chicken, And Spinach Soup _Servings: 4_

Cooking Time: 15 Minutes

Ingredients:

3 tablespoons unsalted butter

2 leeks, white parts only, thinly sliced

4 cups baby spinach

4 cups chicken broth

1 teaspoon salt

¼ teaspoon freshly ground black pepper

2 cups shredded rotisserie chicken

1 tablespoon thinly sliced fresh chives

2 teaspoons grated or minced lemon zest

Directions:

1. Dissolve the butter over high heat in a large pot.

2. Add the leeks and sauté until softened and beginning to brown, 3

to 5 minutes.

3. Add the spinach, broth, salt, and pepper and boil.

4. Simmer within 1 to 2 minutes.

5. Put the chicken and cook within 1 to 2 minutes.

6. Sprinkle with the chives and lemon zest and serve.

Nutrition Info: Calories 256 Total Fat: 12g Total Carbohydrates: 9g Sugar: 3g Fiber: 2g Protein: 27g Sodium: 1483mg

Dark Choco Bombs Servings: 24

Cooking Time: 5 Minutes

Ingredients:

1 cup heavy cream

1 cup cream cheese softened

1 teaspoon vanilla essence

1/2 cup dark chocolate

2 oz. Stevia

Directions:

1. Melt chocolate in a bowl by heating in a microwave.

2. Beat the rest of the ingredients in a mixer until fluffy, then stir in the chocolate melt.

3. Mix well, then divide the mixture in a muffin tray lined with muffin cups.

4. Refrigerate for 3 hrs.

5. Serve.

Nutrition Info: Calories 97 Fat 5 g, Carbs 1 g, Protein 1 g, Fiber 0 g

Italian Stuffed Peppers _Servings: 6_

Cooking Time: 40 Minutes

Ingredients:

1 teaspoon garlic powder

1/2 cup mozzarella, shredded

1 lb. lean ground meat

1/2 cup parmesan cheese

3 bell peppers, cut into half lengthwise, stems, seeds and ribs removed

1 (10 oz.) package frozen spinach

2 cups marinara sauce

1/2 teaspoon salt

1 teaspoon Italian seasoning

Directions:

1. Coat a foil-lined baking sheet with non-stick spray. Place the peppers on the baking pan.

2. Add turkey to a non-stick pan and cook over medium heat until no longer pink.

3. When almost cooked, add 2 cups of marinara sauce and seasonings— Cook for about 8-10 minutes.

4. Add spinach along with 1/2 cup parmesan cheese. Stir until well-combined.

5. Add half cup of the meat mixture into each pepper and divide cheese among all—Preheat the oven to 450 F.

6. Bake peppers for about 25-30 minutes. Cool, and serve.

Nutrition Info: 150 calories 2 g fat 11 g total carbs 20 g protein

Smoked Trout Wrapped In Lettuce _Servings: 4_

Cooking Time: 45 Minutes

Ingredients:

¼ Cup salt-roasted potatoes

1 cup grape tomatoes

½ Cup basil leaves

16 small & medium size lettuce leaves

1/3 cup Asian sweet chili

2 Carrots

1/3 Cup Shallots (thin sliced)

¼ Cup thin slice Jalapenos

1tbsp Sugar

2-4.5 Ounces skinless smoked trout

2tbsp Fresh lime Juice

1 Cucumber

Directions:

1. Cut carrots and cucumber in slim strip size.

2. Marinate these vegetables for 20 mins with sugar, fish sauce, lime juice, shallots, and jalapeno.

3. Add trout pieces and other herbs in this vegetable mixture and blend.

4. Strain water from vegetable and trout mixture and again toss it to blend.

5. Place lettuce leaves on a plate and transfer trout salad on them.

6. Garnish this salad with peanuts and chili sauce.

Nutrition Info: Calories 180 Carbs: 0g Fat: 12g Protein: 18g

Devilled Egg Salad_Ingredients:

12 enormous eggs

1/4 cup slashed green onion

1/2 cup slashed celery

1/2 cup slashed red chime pepper

2 tablespoons Dijon mustard

1/3 cup mayonnaise

1 tablespoon juice, white wine or sherry vinegar 1/4 teaspoon Tabasco or
other hot sauce (pretty much to taste) 1/2 teaspoon paprika (pretty much to
taste) 1/2 teaspoon dark pepper (pretty much to taste) 1/4 teaspoon salt
(more to taste)

Directions:

1. Hard heat up the eggs: The simplest method to make hard bubbled eggs
that are anything but difficult to strip is to steam them.

Fill a pan with 1 inch of water and addition a steamer bushel. (On the off
chance that you don't have a steamer bushel, that is alright.) 2. Heat the
water to the point of boiling, delicately place the eggs in the steamer bin or
straightforwardly in the pan. Spread the pot. Set your clock for 15 minutes.
Evacuate eggs and set in frigid virus water to cool.

3. Prep the eggs and veggies: Chop the eggs coarsely and put them into a huge bowl. Include the green onion, celery, and red chime pepper.

4. Make the plate of mixed greens: In little bowl, combine the mayo, mustard, vinegar, and Tabasco. Tenderly mix the mayo dressing into the bowl with the eggs and vegetables. Include the paprika and salt and dark pepper. Change seasonings to taste.

Sesame-tamari Baked Chicken With Green Beans

Servings: 4

Cooking Time: 45 Minutes

Ingredients:

1-pound green beans, trimmed

4 bone-in, skin-on chicken breasts

2 tablespoons honey

1 tablespoon sesame oil

1 tablespoon gluten-free tamari or soy sauce 1 cup chicken or vegetable broth

Directions:

1. Preheat the oven to 400°F.

2. Arrange the green beans on a large rimmed baking sheet.

3. Put the chicken, skin-side up, on top of the beans.

4. Drizzle with the honey, oil, and tamari. Add the broth.

5. Roast within 35 to 40 minutes. Remove, let it rest for 5 minutes and serve.

Nutrition Info: Calories 378 Total Fat: 10g Total Carbohydrates: 19g Sugar: 10g Fiber: 4g Protein: 54g Sodium: 336mg

Ginger Chicken Stew *Servings: 6*

Cooking Time: 20 Minutes

Ingredients:

¼ cup chicken thigh fillet, diced

¼ cup cooked egg noodles

1 unripe papaya, peeled, diced

1 cup chicken broth, low-sodium, low-fat

1 medallion ginger, peeled, crushed

dash onion powder

dash garlic powder, add more if desired

1 cup of water

1 tsp. fish sauce

dash white pepper

1-piece, small bird's eye chili, minced

Directions:

1. Put all the fixing in a large Dutch oven set over high heat. Boil.

Turn down heat to the lowest setting. Put the lid on.

2. Let the stew cook for 20 minutes or until papaya is fork-tender.

Turn off heat. Consume as is, or with ½ cup of cooked rice. Serve warm.

Nutrition Info: Calories 273 Carbs: 15g Fat: 9g Protein: 33g

Creamy Garbano Salad Ingredients:

Plate of mixed greens

2 14 oz jars Chickpeas

3/4 cup Carrot little shakers

3/4 cup Celery little shakers

3/4 cup Bell Pepper Small shakers

1 Scallion hacked

1/4 cup Red Onion little shakers

1/2 Large Avocado

6 oz smooth tofu

1 Tbsp Apple Cider Vinegar

1 Tbsp Lemon Juice

1 Tbsp Dijon Mustard

1 Tbsp Sweet Relish

1/4 tsp Smoked Paprika

1/4 tsp Celery seeds

1/4 tsp Black Pepper

1/4 tsp Mustard powder

Ocean salt to taste

Sandwich Fix'ns

Grown Whole Grain Bread

Cut Roma Tomatoes

Spread Lettuce

Directions:

1. Get ready and slash your carrots, celery, chime pepper, red onion and scallion and spot in a little blending bowl. Put In a safe spot.

2. Utilizing a little submersion blender or nourishment processor, mix the avocado, tofu, apple juice vinegar, lemon juice, and mustard until smooth.

3. Strain and wash your garbanzos, and spot in a medium blending bowl. With a potato masher or a fork squash the beans until most are separated and it begins to take after fish plate of mixed greens. You don't need it to be smooth however finished and stout. Season the beans with a spot of salt and pepper.

4. Include the cleaved vegetables, avocado-tofu cream, and the rest of the flavors and relish and blend well. Taste and alter as indicated by your inclination.

Carrot Noodles With Ginger Lime Peanut Sauce

Ingredients:

For the carrot pasta:

5 huge carrots, stripped and julienned or spiraled into slim strips 1/3 cup (50g) cooked cashews

2 tablespoons new cilantro, finely hacked

For the ginger-peanut sauce:

2 tablespoons rich nutty spread

4 tablespoons ordinary coconut milk

Squeeze cayenne pepper

2 huge cloves garlic, finely hacked

1 tablespoon new ginger, stripped and ground 1 tablespoon lime juice

Salt, to taste

Directions:

1. Consolidate all sauce ingredients in a little bowl and combine until smooth and rich and put in a safe spot while you julienne/spiralize the carrots.

2. In a huge serving bowl, tenderly hurl the carrots and sauce together until equally covered. Top with broiled cashews (or peanuts) and newly hacked cilantro.

Roasted Vegetables With Sweet Potatoes And White Beans

Servings: 4

Cooking Time: 25 Minutes

Ingredients:

2 small sweet potatoes, dice

½ red onion, cut into ¼-inch dice

1 medium carrot, peeled and thinly sliced

4 ounces green beans, trimmed

¼ cup extra-virgin olive oil

1 teaspoon salt

¼ teaspoon freshly ground black pepper

1 (15½-ounce) can white beans, drained and rinsed 1 tablespoon minced or grated lemon zest

1 tablespoon chopped fresh dill

Directions:

1. Preheat the oven to 400°F.

2. Combine the sweet potatoes, onion, carrot, green beans, oil, salt, and pepper on a large rimmed baking sheet and mix to combine well. Arrange in a single layer.

3. Roast until the vegetables are tender, 20 to 25 minutes.

4. Add the white beans, lemon zest, and dill, mix well and serve.

Nutrition Info: Calories 315 Total Fat: 13g Total Carbohydrates: 42g Sugar: 5g Fiber: 13g Protein: 10g Sodium: 632mg

Kale Salad <u>*Servings: 1*</u>

Cooking Time: 0 Minutes

Ingredients:

1 cup of fresh kale

½ cup of blueberries

½ cup of pitted cherries halved

¼ cup of dried cranberries

1 tablespoon of sesame seeds

2 tablespoons of olive oil

Juice of 1 lemon

Directions:

1. Combine the olive oil and lemon juice, then toss the kale in the dressing.

2. Put the kale leaves into a salad bowl, and top with the fresh blueberries, cherries, and cranberries.

3. Top with the sesame seeds.

<u>Nutrition Info:</u> Total Carbohydrates 48g Dietary Fiber: 7g Protein: 6g Total Fat: 33g Calories: 477

Coconut And Hazelnut Chilled Glass <u>Servings: 1</u>

Cooking Time: 0 Minute

Ingredients:

½ cup coconut almond milk

¼ cup hazelnuts, chopped

1 and ½ cups water

1 pack stevia

Directions:

1. Add listed Ingredients to the blender

2. Blend until you have a smooth and creamy texture 3. Serve chilled and enjoy!

<u>Nutrition Info:</u> Calories: 457Fat: 46gCarbohydrates: 12gProtein: 7g

Cool Garbanzo And Spinach Beans _Servings: 4_

Cooking Time: 0 Minute

Ingredients:

1 tablespoon olive oil

½ onion, diced

10 ounces spinach, chopped

12 ounces garbanzo beans

½ teaspoon cumin

Directions:

1. Take a skillet and add olive oil, let it warm over medium-low heat 2. Add onions, garbanzo and cook for 5 minutes 3. Stir in spinach, cumin, garbanzo beans and season with salt 4. Use a spoon to smash gently

5. Cook thoroughly until heated, enjoy!

Nutrition Info: Calories: 90Fat: 4gCarbohydrates: 11gProtein: 4g

Taro Leaves In Coconut Sauce _Servings: 5_

Cooking Time: 20 Minutes

Ingredients:

4 cups dried taro leaves

2 cans of coconut cream, divided

¼ cup ground pork, 90% lean

1 tsp. shrimp paste

1 bird's eye chili, minced

Directions:

1. Except for 1 can of coconut cream, place all ingredients in a crockpot set at medium setting. Secure lid. Cook undisturbed for 3 to 3½ hours.

2. Pour the remaining can of coconut cream before turning off the heat. Stir and serve.

Nutrition Info: Calories 264 Carbs: 8g Fat: 24g Protein: 4g

Roasted Tofu And Greens _Servings: 4_

Cooking Time: 20 Minutes

Ingredients:

3 cups baby spinach or kale

1 tablespoon sesame oil

1 tablespoon ginger, minced

1 garlic clove, minced

1-pound firm tofu, cut into 1-inch dice

1 tablespoon gluten-free tamari or soy sauce ¼ teaspoon red pepper flakes (optional)

1 teaspoon rice vinegar

2 scallions, thinly sliced

Directions:

1. Preheat the oven to 400°F.

2. Combine the spinach, oil, ginger, and garlic on a large rimmed baking sheet.

3. Bake until the spinach has wilted, 3 to 5 minutes.

4. Add the tofu, tamari, and red pepper flakes (if using) and toss to combine well.

5. Bake until the tofu is beginning to brown, 10 to 15 minutes.

6. Top with the vinegar and scallions and serve.

Nutrition Info: Calories 121 Total Fat: 8g Total Carbohydrates: 4g Sugar: 1g Fiber: 2g Protein: 10g Sodium: 258mg

Spiced Broccoli, Cauliflower, And Tofu With Red Onion

Servings: 2

Cooking Time: 25 Minutes

Ingredients:

2 cups broccoli florets

2 cups cauliflower florets

1 medium red onion, diced

3 tablespoons extra-virgin olive oil

1 teaspoon salt

¼ teaspoon freshly ground black pepper

1-pound firm tofu, cut into 1-inch dice

1 garlic clove, minced

1 (¼-inch) piece fresh ginger, minced

Directions:

1. Preheat the oven to 400°F.

2. Combine the broccoli, cauliflower, onion, oil, salt, and pepper on a large rimmed baking sheet, and mix well.

3. Roast until the vegetables have softened, 10 to 15 minutes.

4. Add the tofu, garlic, and ginger. Roast within 10 minutes.

5. Gently mix the ingredients on the baking sheet to combine the tofu with the vegetables and serve.

Nutrition Info: Calories 210 Total Fat: 15g Total Carbohydrates: 11g Sugar: 4g Fiber: 4g Protein: 12g Sodium: 626mg

Beans And Salmon Pan _Servings: 4_

Cooking Time: 25 Minutes

Ingredients:

1 cup canned black beans, drained and rinsed 4 garlic cloves, minced

1 yellow onion, chopped

2 tablespoons olive oil

4 salmon fillets, boneless

½ teaspoon coriander, ground

1 teaspoon turmeric powder

2 tomatoes, cubed

½ cup chicken stock

A pinch of salt and black pepper

½ teaspoon cumin seeds

1 tablespoon chives, chopped

Directions:

1. Heat up a pan with the oil over medium heat, add the onion and the garlic and sauté for 5 minutes.

2. Add the fish and sear it for 2 minutes on each side.

3. Add the beans and the other ingredients, toss gently and cook for 10 minutes more.

4. Divide the mix between plates and serve right away for lunch.

Nutrition Info: calories 219, fat 8, fiber 8, carbs 12, protein 8

Carrot Soup Servings: 4

Cooking Time: 40 Minutes

Ingredients:

1 cup Butternut Squash, chopped

1 tbsp. Olive Oil

1 tbsp. Turmeric Powder

14 ½ oz. Coconut Milk, light

3 cups Carrot, chopped

1 Leek, rinsed & sliced

1 tbsp. Ginger, grated

3 cups Vegetable Broth

1 cup Fennel, chopped

Salt & Pepper, to taste

2 cloves of Garlic, minced

Directions:

1. Start by heating a Dutch oven over medium-high heat.

2. To this, spoon in the oil and then stir in fennel, squash, carrots, and leek. Mix well.

3. Now, sauté it for 4 to 5 minutes or until softened.

4. Next, add turmeric, ginger, pepper, and garlic to it. Cook for another 1 to 2 minutes.

5. Then, pour the broth and coconut milk to it. Combine well.

6. After that, bring the mixture to a boil and cover the Dutch oven.

7. Allow it to simmer for 20 minutes.

8. Once cooked, transfer the mixture to a high-speed blender and blend for 1 to 2 minutes or until you get a creamy smooth soup.

9. Check for seasoning and spoon in more salt and pepper if needed.

Nutrition Info: Calories: 210.4KcalProteins: 2.11gCarbohydrates: 25.64gFat: 10.91g

Healthy Pasta Salad <u>*Servings: 6*</u>

Cooking Time: 10 Minutes

Ingredients:

1 package of gluten-free fusilli pasta

1 cup of grape tomatoes, sliced

1 handful of fresh cilantro, chopped

1 cup of olives, halved

1 cup of fresh basil, chopped

½ cup of olive oil

Sea salt to taste

Directions:

1. Whisk together the olive oil, chopped basil, cilantro, and sea salt.

Set aside.

2. Cook the pasta according to package directions, strain, and rinse.

3. Combine the pasta with the tomatoes and olives.

4. Add the olive oil mixture, and toss until well combined.

<u>Nutrition Info:</u> Total Carbohydrates 66g Dietary Fiber: 5g Protein: 13g Total Fat: 23g Calories: 525

Chickpea Curry _Servings: 4 To 6_

Cooking Time: 25 Minutes

Ingredients:

2 × 15 oz. Chickpeas, washed, drained & cooked 2 tbsp. Olive Oil

1 tbsp. Turmeric Powder

½ of 1 Onion, diced

1 tsp. Cayenne, grounded

4 Garlic cloves, minced

2 tsp. Chili Powder

15 oz. Tomato Puree

Black Pepper, as needed

2 tbsp. Tomato Paste

1 tsp. Cayenne, grounded

½ tbsp. Maple Syrup

½ of 15 oz. can of Coconut Milk

2 tsp. Cumin, grounded

2 tsp. Smoked Paprika

Directions:

1. Heat a large skillet over medium-high heat. To this, spoon in the oil.

2. Once the oil becomes hot, stir in the onion and cook for 3 to 4

minutes or until softened.

3. Next, spoon in the tomato paste, maple syrup, all seasonings, tomato puree, and garlic into it. Mix well.

4. Then, add the cooked chickpeas to it along with coconut milk, black pepper, and salt.

5. Now, give everything a good stir and allow it to simmer for 8 to 10

minutes or until thickened.

6. Drizzle lime juice over it and garnish with cilantro, if desired.

Nutrition Info: Calories: 224KcalProteins: 15.2gCarbohydrates: 32.4gFat: 7.5g

Ground Meat Stroganoff_Ingredients:

1 lb lean ground meat

1 little onion diced

1 clove garlic minced

3/4 lb new mushrooms cut

3 tablespoons flour

2 cups meat stock

salt and pepper to taste

2 teaspoons Worcestershire sauce

3/4 cup sharp cream

2 tablespoons new parsley

Directions:

1. Dark colored ground hamburger, onion and garlic (making an effort not to split it up something over the top) in a dish until no pink remains. Channel fat.

2. Include cut mushrooms and cook 2-3 minutes. Mix in flour and cook 1 progressively minute.

3. Include stock, Worcestershire sauce, salt and pepper and heat to the point of boiling. Lessen warmth and stew on low 10 minutes.

Cook egg noodles as indicated by bundle headings.

4. Expel meat blend from the warmth, mix in sharp cream and parsley.

5. Serve over egg noodles.

Saucy Short Ribs _Servings: 4_

Cooking Time: 65 Minutes

Ingredients:

2 lbs. beef short ribs

1 ½ tsp olive oil

1 ½ tbsp soy sauce

1 tbsp Worcestershire sauce

1 tbsp stevia

1 ¼ cups onion chopped.

1 tsp garlic minced

1/2 cup red wine

⅓ cup ketchup, sugar-free

Salt and black pepper to taste

Directions:

1. Slice the ribs into 3 segments and rub them with black pepper and salt.

2. Add oil to the Instant Pot and hit Sauté.

3. Place the ribs in the oil and sear for 5 minutes per side.

4. Toss in onion and sauté for 4 minutes.

5. Stir in garlic and cook for 1 minute.

6. Whisk rest of the ingredients in a bowl and pour over the ribs.

7. Put on its pressure lid and cook for 55 minutes on Manual mode at High pressure.

8. Once done, release the pressure naturally then remove the lid.

9. Serve warm.

Nutrition Info: Calories 555, Carbs 12.8g, Protein 66.7g, Fat 22.3g, Fiber 0.9g

Chicken And Gluten-free Noodle Soup *Servings:* *4*

Cooking Time: 25 Minutes

Ingredients:

¼ cup extra-virgin olive oil

3 celery stalks, cut into ¼-inch slices

2 medium carrots, cut into ¼-inch dice

1 small onion, cut into ¼-inch dice

1 fresh rosemary sprig

4 cups chicken broth

8 ounces gluten-free penne

1 teaspoon salt

¼ teaspoon freshly ground black pepper

2 cups diced rotisserie chicken

¼ cup finely chopped fresh flat-leaf parsley Directions:

1. Heat-up the oil over high heat in a large pot.

2. Put the celery, carrots, onion, and rosemary and sauté until softened, 5 to 7 minutes.

3. Add the broth, penne, salt, and pepper and boil.

4. Simmer and cook until the penne is tender, 8 to 10 minutes.

5. Remove and discard the rosemary sprig, and add the chicken and parsley.

6. Reduce the heat to low. Cook within 5 minutes, and serve.

Nutrition Info: Calories 485 Total Fat: 18g Total Carbohydrates: 47g Sugar: 4g Fiber: 7g Protein: 33g Sodium: 1423mg

Lentil Curry _Servings: 4_

Cooking Time: 40 Minutes

Ingredients:

2 tsp. Mustard Seeds

1 tsp. Turmeric, grounded

1 cup Lentils, soaked

2 tsp. Cumin Seeds

1 Tomato, large & chopped

1 Yellow Onion, sliced finely

4 cups Water

Sea Salt, as needed

2 Carrots, sliced into half-moons

3 handful of Spinach leaves, shredded

1 tsp. Ginger, minced

½ tsp. Chili Powder

2 tbsp. Coconut Oil

Directions:

1. First, place the mung beans and water in a deep saucepan over medium-high heat.

2. Now, bring the beans mixture to a boil and allow it to simmer.

3. Simmer within 20 to 30 minutes or until the mung beans are softened.

4. Then, heat the coconut oil in a large saucepan over medium heat and stir in the mustard seeds and cumin seeds.

5. If the mustard seeds pop, put the onions. Sauté the onions for 4

minutes or until they softened.

6. Spoon in the garlic and continue sautéing for another 1 minute.

Once aromatic, spoon in the turmeric and chili powder to it.

7. Then, add the carrot and tomato—Cook for 6 minutes or until softened.

8. Finally, add the cooked lentils to it and give everything a good stir.

9. Stir in the spinach leaves and sauté until wilted. Remove from heat. Serve it warm and enjoy.

Nutrition Info: Calories 290Kcal Proteins: 14g Carbohydrates: 43g Fat: 8g

Chicken And Snap Pea Stir-fry _Servings: 4_

Cooking Time: 10 Minutes

Ingredients:

1 ¼ cups boneless skinless chicken breast, thinly sliced 3 tablespoons fresh cilantro, chopped

2 tablespoons vegetable oil

2 tablespoons of sesame seeds

1 bunch scallions, thinly sliced

2 teaspoons Sriracha

2 garlic cloves, minced

2 tablespoons rice vinegar

1 bell pepper, thinly sliced

3 tablespoons soy sauce

2½ cups snap peas

Salt, to taste

Freshly ground black pepper, to taste

Directions:

1. Heat-up the oil in a pan over medium heat. Add garlic and thinly sliced scallions. Cook for a minute and then add 2 ½ cups snap peas along with bell pepper. Cook until tender, just for about 3-4 minutes.

2. Add chicken and cook for about 4-5 minutes, or until thoroughly cooked.

3. Add in 2 teaspoons Sriracha, 2 tablespoons of sesame seeds, 3

tablespoons soy sauce, and 2 tablespoons rice vinegar. Toss everything until well-combined. Simmer within 2-3 minutes over low heat.

4. Add 3 tablespoons of chopped cilantro and stir well. Transfer, and sprinkle with extra sesame seeds and cilantro, if needed. Enjoy!

Nutrition Info: 228 calories 11 g fat 11 g total carbs 20 g protein

Juicy Broccolini With Anchovy Almonds

Servings: 6

Cooking Time: 10 Minutes

Ingredients:

2 bunches of broccolini, trimmed

1 tablespoon extra-virgin olive oil

1 long fresh red chili, deseeded, finely chopped 2 garlic cloves, thinly sliced

¼ cup natural almonds, coarsely chopped

2 teaspoons lemon rind, finely grated

A squeeze of lemon juice, fresh

4 anchovies in oil, chopped

Directions:

1. Warm the oil until hot in a large saucepan. Add the drained anchovies, garlic, chili, and lemon rind. Cook until aromatic, for 30

seconds, stirring frequently. Add the almond & continue to cook for a minute more, stirring frequently. Remove from the heat & add a squeeze of fresh lemon juice.

2. Then place the broccolini in a steamer basket set over a saucepan of simmering water. Cover & cook until crisp-tender, for 2

to 3 minutes. Drain well and then transfer to a large-sized serving plate. Top with the almond mixture. Enjoy.

Nutrition Info: kcal 350 Fat: 7 g Fiber: 3 g Protein: 6 g

Shiitake And Spinach Pattie Servings: 8

Cooking Time: 15 Minutes

Ingredients:

1 ½ cups shiitake mushrooms, minced

1 ½ cups spinach, chopped

3 garlic cloves, minced

2 onions, minced

4 tsp. olive oil

1 egg

1 ½ cups quinoa, cooked

1 ½ tsp. Italian seasoning

1/3 cup toasted sunflower seeds, ground

1/3 cup Pecorino cheese, grated

Directions:

1. Heat olive oil in a saucepan. Once hot, sauté shiitake mushrooms for 3 minutes or until lightly seared. Add in garlic and onion. Sauté for 2 minutes or until fragrant and translucent. Set aside.

2. In the same saucepan, heat the remaining olive oil. Add in spinach. Reduce heat, then simmer for 1 minute, drain and transfer to a strainer.

3. Chop spinach finely and add into the mushroom mixture. Add egg into the spinach mixture. Fold in cooked quinoa—season with Italian seasoning, then mix until well combined. Sprinkle sunflower seeds and cheese.

4. Divide the spinach mixture into patties—Cook patties within 5

minutes or until firm and golden brown. Serve with burger bread.

Nutrition Info: Calories 43 Carbs: 9g Fat: 0g Protein: 3g

Broccoli Cauliflower Salad _Servings: 6_

Cooking Time: 20 Minutes

Ingredients:

¼ tsp. Black Pepper, grounded

3 cups Cauliflower Florets

1 tbsp. Vinegar

1 tsp. Honey

8 cups Kale, chopped

3 cups Broccoli Florets

4 tbsp. Extra Virgin Olive Oil

½ tsp. Salt

1 ½ tsp. Dijon Mustard

1 tsp. Honey

½ cup Cherries, dried

1/3 cup Pecans, chopped

1 cup Manchego cheese, shaved

Directions:

1. Preheat the oven to 450 ° F and place a baking sheet in the middle rack.

2. After that, place cauliflower and broccoli florets in a large bowl.

3. To this, spoon in half of the salt, two tablespoons of the oil and pepper. Toss well.

4. Now, transfer the mixture to the preheated sheet and bake it for 12 minutes while flipping it once in between.

5. Once it becomes tender and golden in color, remove it from the oven and allow it to cool completely.

6. In the meantime, mix the remaining two tablespoons of oil, vinegar, honey, mustard, and salt in another bowl.

7. Brush this mixture over the kale leaves by messaging the leaves with your hands. Set it aside for 3 to 5 minutes.

8. Finally, stir in the roasted vegetables, cheese, cherries, and pecan to the broccoli-cauliflower salad.

Nutrition Info: Calories: 259KcalProteins: 8.4gCarbohydrates: 23.2gFat: 16.3g

Chicken Salad With Chinese Touch *Servings: 3*

Cooking Time: 25 Minutes

Ingredients:

1 Medium green onion (thinly sliced)

2 Boneless chicken breasts

2tbsp Soya sauce

¼ Teaspoon white pepper

1tbsp sesame oil

4 cups romaine lettuce (chopped)

1 cup cabbage (shredded)

¼ Cup small cubes carrots

¼ Cup thin sliced almonds

¼ Cup noodles (only for serving)

For Preparing Chinese Dressing:

1 Minced garlic clove

1 Teaspoon soy sauce

1tbsp sesame oil

2tbsp Rice vinegar

1tbsp Sugar

Directions:

1. Prepare Chinese dressing by whisking all ingredients in a bowl.

2. In a bowl, marinate chicken breasts with garlic, olive oil, soy sauce, and white pepper for 20 minutes.

3. Place baking dish in the preheated oven (at 225C).

4. Place chicken breasts in the baking dish and bake it almost for 20

minutes.

5. For assembling the salad, combine romaine lettuce, cabbage, carrots, and green onion.

6. For serving, place a chicken piece in a plate and salad on top of it. Pour some dressing over it alongside noodles.

Nutrition Info: Calories 130 Carbs: 10g Fat: 6g Protein: 10g

Amaranth And Quinoa Stuffed Peppers

Servings: 4

Cooking Time: 1 Hour & 10 Minutes

Ingredients:

2 tablespoons Amaranth

1 medium zucchini, trimmed, grated

2 vine-ripened tomatoes, diced

2/3 cup (approximately 135 g) quinoa

1 onion, medium-sized, chopped finely

2 crushed garlic cloves

1 teaspoon ground cumin

2 tablespoons lightly toasted sunflower seeds 75g ricotta cheese, fresh

2 tablespoons currants

4 capsicums, large, halved lengthwise & seeded 2 tablespoons flat-leaf parsley, roughly chopped Directions:

1. Line a baking tray, preferably large-sized with some baking paper (nonstick) and then preheat your oven to 350 F in advance. Fill a medium-

sized saucepan with an approximately a half-liter of water and then add the amaranth and quinoa; bring it to a boil over moderate heat. Once done, decrease the heat to low; cover & let simmer until grains turn al dente and water is absorbed, for 12 to 15

minutes. Remove from the heat & set aside.

2. In the meantime, lightly coat a large-sized frying pan with oil and heat it over medium heat. Once hot, add the onion with zucchini & cook until softened, for a couple of minutes, stirring frequently. Add the cumin and garlic; cook for a minute. Remove from the heat & set aside to cool.

3. Place the grains, onion mixture, sunflower seeds, currants, parsley, ricotta, and tomato in a mixing bowl, preferably large-sized; give the ingredients a good stir until combined well—season with pepper and salt to taste.

4. Fill the capsicums with prepared quinoa mixture & arrange them on the tray, covering the tray with aluminum foil—Bake for 17 to 20

minutes. Remove the foil & bake until the stuffing turns into golden & vegetables turn fork-tender, for 15 to 20 more minutes.

Nutrition Info: kcal 200 Fat: 8.5 g Fiber: 8 g Protein: 15 g

Crispy Cheese-crusted Fish Fillet _Servings: 4_

Cooking Time: 10 Minutes

Ingredients:

¼-cup whole-wheat breadcrumbs

¼-cup Parmesan cheese, grated

¼-tsp sea salt ¼-tsp ground pepper

1-Tbsp. olive oil 4-pcs tilapia fillets

Directions:

1. Preheat the oven to 375°F.

2. Stir in the breadcrumbs, Parmesan cheese, salt, pepper, and olive oil in a mixing bowl.

3. Mix well until blended thoroughly.

4. Coat the fillets with the mixture, and lay each on a lightly sprayed baking sheet.

5. Place the sheet in the oven.

6. Bake for 10 minutes until the fillets cook through and turn brownish.

<u>Nutrition Info:</u> Calories: 255Fat: 7gProtein: 15.9gCarbs: 34gFiber: 2.6g

Protein Power Beans And Green Stuffed_Shells

Ingredients:

Genuine or ocean salt

Olive oil

12 oz. bundle kind sized shells (around 40) 1 lb. solidified cleaved spinach

2 to 3 cloves garlic, stripped and divided

15 to 16 oz. ricotta cheddar (ideally full fat/entire milk) 2 eggs

1 can white beans, (for example, cannellini), depleted and flushed

½ C green pesto, custom made or locally acquired Ground dark pepper

3 C (or more) marinara sauce

Ground parmesan or pecorino cheddar (discretionary) <u>Directions:</u>

1. Heat at any rate 5 quarts of water to the point of boiling in an enormous pot (or work in two littler clumps). Include a tablespoon of salt, a sprinkle of olive oil, and the shells. Bubble around 9 minutes (or until extremely still somewhat firm), blending sporadically to keep the shells isolated. Tenderly channel the shells in a colander, or scoop from the water with an opened spoon. Wash quickly with cool water. Line a rimmed heating sheet with cling wrap. At the point when the shells are sufficiently cool to deal with,

separate them by hand, dumping out extra water and putting opening up in a solitary layer on the sheet container. Spread with progressively plastic wrap once practically cool.

2. Bring a couple of quarts of water (or utilize remaining pasta water, on the off chance that you didn't dump it out) to a bubble in a similar pot. Include solidified spinach and cook three minutes on high, until delicate. Line the colander with soggy paper towels on the off chance that the openings are enormous, at that point channel the spinach. Set colander over a bowl to deplete more while you start the filling.

3. Add only the garlic to a nourishment processor and run until it's finely hacked and adhering to the sides. Scratch down the sides of the bowl, at that point include the ricotta, eggs, beans, pesto, 1½

teaspoons salt, and a few toils of pepper (a major squeeze). Press the spinach in your grasp to deplete well of outstanding water, at that point add to different fixings in the nourishment processor. Run until practically smooth, with a couple of little bits of spinach still noticeable. I lean toward not to taste subsequent to including the crude egg, yet on the off chance that you think that its fundamental taste a little and modify flavoring to taste.

4. Preheat the broiler to 350 (F) and shower or gently oil a 9 x 13"

skillet, in addition to another littler goulash dish (around 8 to 10 of the shells won't fit in the 9 x 13). To fill the shells, get each shell in turn, holding it open with thumb and pointer finger of your non-predominant hand.

Scoop 3 to 4 tablespoons loading up with your other hand and scratch into the shell. The greater part of them won't look great, which is alright! Spot filled shells near one another in the readied container. Spoon sauce over the shells, leaving bits of the green filling unmistakable. Spread container with thwart and prepare for 30 minutes. Increment warmth to 375 (F), sprinkle shells with some ground parmesan (if utilizing), and heat revealed for another 5

to 10 minutes until cheddar is dissolved and abundance dampness is diminished.

5. Cool 5 to 10 minutes, at that point serve alone or with a fresh plate of mixed greens as an afterthought!

Asian Noodle Salad Ingredients:

8 ounces in length slight entire wheat pasta noodles —, for example, spaghetti (use soba noodles to make gluten free) 24 ounces Mann's Broccoli Cole Slaw — 2 12-ounce sacks 4 ounces ground carrots

1/4 cup extra-virgin olive oil

1/4 cup rice vinegar

3 tablespoons nectar — utilize light agave nectar to make veggie lover

3 tablespoons smooth nutty spread

2 tablespoons low-sodium soy sauce — gluten free if necessary 1 tablespoon Sriracha pepper sauce — or garlic chile sauce, in addition to extra to taste

1 tablespoon minced new ginger

2 teaspoons minced garlic — around 4 cloves 3/4 cup broiled unsalted peanuts, — generally slashed 3/4 cup new cilantro — finely slashed

Directions:

1. Heat a huge pot of salted water to the point of boiling. Cook the noodles until still somewhat firm, as per bundle headings. Channel and flush quickly with cool water to evacuate the overabundance starch and stop the

cooking, at that point move to a huge serving bowl. Include the broccoli cole slaw and carrots.

2. While the pasta cooks, whisk together the olive oil, rice vinegar, nectar, nutty spread, soy sauce, Sriarcha, ginger, and garlic. Pour over the noodle blend and hurl to consolidate. Include the peanuts and cilantro and hurl again. Serve chilled or at room temperature with extra Sriracha sauce as wanted.

3. Formula Notes

4. Asian Noodle Salad can be served cold or at room temperature.

Store remains in the cooler in a water/air proof holder for as long as 3 days.

Salmon And Green Beans _Servings: 4_

Cooking Time: 26 Minutes

Ingredients:

2 tablespoons olive oil

1 yellow onion, chopped

4 salmon fillets, boneless

1 cup green beans, trimmed and halved

2 garlic cloves, minced

½ cup chicken stock

1 teaspoon chili powder

1 teaspoon sweet paprika

A pinch of salt and black pepper

1 tablespoon cilantro, chopped

Directions:

1. Heat up a pan with the oil over medium heat, add onion, stir and sauté for 2 minutes.

2. Add the fish and sear it for 2 minutes on each side.

3. Add the rest of the ingredients, toss gently and bake everything at 360 degrees F for 20 minutes.

4. Divide everything between plates and serve for lunch.

Nutrition Info: calories 322, fat 18.3, fiber 2, carbs 5.8, protein 35.7

Cheesy Stuffed Chicken_Ingredients:

2 scallions (meagerly cut)

2 seeded jalapeños (meagerly cut)

1/4 c. cilantro

1 tsp. lime pizzazz

4 oz. Monterey Jack cheddar (coarsely ground) 4 little boneless, skinless chicken bosoms

3 tbsp. olive oil

Salt

Pepper

3 tbsp. lime juice

2 ringer peppers (daintily cut)

1/2 little red onion (meagerly cut)

5 c. torn romaine lettuce

Directions:

1. Warmth broiler to 450°F. In bowl, consolidate scallions and seeded jalapeños, 1/4 cup cilantro (cleaved) and lime get-up-and-go, at that point hurl with Monterey Jack cheddar.

2. Supplement blade into thickest piece of every one of boneless, skinless chicken bosoms and move to and fro to make 2 1/2-inch pocket that is as wide as conceivable without experiencing. Stuff chicken with cheddar blend.

3. Warmth 2 tablespoons olive oil in enormous skillet on medium.

Season chicken with salt and pepper and cook until brilliant darker on 1 side, 3 to 4 minutes. Turn chicken over and broil until cooked through, 10 to 12 minutes.

4. In the interim, in huge bowl, whisk together lime juice, 1

tablespoon olive oil and 1/2 teaspoon salt. Include ringer peppers and red onion and let sit 10 minutes, hurling sporadically. Hurl with romaine lettuce and 1 cup new cilantro. Present with chicken and lime wedges.

Arugula With Gorgonzola Dressing <u>Servings: 4</u>

Cooking Time: 0 Minutes

Ingredients:

1 bunch of arugulas, cleaned

1 pear, sliced thinly

1 tablespoon fresh lemon juice

1 garlic clove, bruised

1/3 cup Gorgonzola cheese, crumbled

1/4 cup vegetable stock, reduced-sodium

Freshly ground pepper

4 teaspoons olive oil

1 tablespoon of cider vinegar

Directions:

1. Put the pear slices and lemon juice in a bowl. Toss to coat.

Arrange the pear slices, along with the arugula, on a platter.

2. In a bowl, combine the vinegar, oil, cheese, broth, pepper, and garlic. Leave for 5 minutes, remove the garlic. Put the dressing, then serve.

Nutrition Info: Calories 145 Carbs: 23g Fat: 4g Protein: 6g

Cabbage Soup _Servings: 6_

Cooking Time: 35 Minutes

Ingredients:

1 yellow onion, chopped

1 green cabbage head, shredded

2 tablespoons olive oil

5 cups veggie stock

1 carrot, peeled and grated

A pinch of salt and black pepper

1 tablespoon cilantro, chopped

2 teaspoons thyme, chopped

½ teaspoon smoked paprika

½ teaspoon hot paprika

1 tablespoon lemon juice

Cauliflower Rice *Servings: 4*

Cooking Time: 10 Minutes

Ingredients:

¼ cup Cooking Oil

1 tbsp. Coconut Oil

1 tbsp. Coconut Sugar

4 cups Cauliflower, broken down into florets ½ tsp. Salt

Directions:

1. First, process the cauliflower in a food processor and process it for 1 to 2 minutes.

2. Heat-up the oil in a large skillet over medium heat, then spoon in the riced cauliflower, coconut sugar, and salt to the pan.

3. Combine them well and cook them for 4 to 5 minutes or until the cauliflower is slightly soft.

4. Finally, pour the coconut milk and enjoy it.

Nutrition Info: Calories 108Kcal Proteins:27.1g Carbohydrates: 11g Fat: 6g

Feta Frittata & Spinach Servings: 4

Cooking Time: 10 Minutes

Ingredients:

½ small brown onion

250g baby spinach

½ cup feta cheese

1 tbsp garlic paste

4 beaten eggs

Seasoning Mix

Salt & Pepper according to taste

1 tbsp olive oil

Directions:

1. Add finely chop an onion in oil and cook it on medium flame.

2. Add spinach in light brown onions and toss it for 2 min.

3. In eggs, add the mixture of cold spinach and onions.

4. Now add garlic paste, salt, and pepper and mix the mixture.

5. Cook this mixture on low flame and stir eggs gently.

6. Add feta cheese on the eggs and place the pan under the already preheat grill.

7. Cook it almost for 2 to 3 minutes until the frittata is brown.

8. Serve this feta frittata hot or cold.

Nutrition Info: Calories 210 Carbs: 5g Fat: 14g Protein: 21g

Fiery Chicken Pot Stickers_Ingredients:

1-pound ground chicken

1/2 cup destroyed cabbage

1 carrot, stripped and destroyed

2 cloves garlic, squeezed

2 green onions, meagerly cut

1 tablespoon diminished sodium soy sauce

1 tablespoon hoisin sauce

1 tablespoon naturally ground ginger

2 teaspoons sesame oil

1/4 teaspoon ground white pepper

36 won ton wrappers

2 tablespoons vegetable oil

FOR THE HOT CHILI OIL SAUCE:

1/2 cup vegetable oil

1/4 cup dried red chillies, squashed

2 cloves garlic, minced

Directions:

1. Warmth vegetable oil in a little pan over medium warmth. Mix in squashed peppers and garlic, mixing every so often, until the oil arrives at 180 degrees F, around 8-10 minutes; put in a safe spot.

2. In an enormous bowl, join chicken, cabbage, carrot, garlic, green onions, soy sauce, hoisin sauce, ginger, sesame oil and white pepper.

3. To collect the dumplings, place wrappers on a work surface.

Spoon 1 tablespoon of the chicken blend into the focal point of every wrapper. Utilizing your finger, rub the edges of the wrappers with water. Crease the mixture over the filling to make a half-moon shape, squeezing the edges to seal.

4. Warmth vegetable oil in a huge skillet over medium warmth.

Include pot stickers in a solitary layer and cook until brilliant and fresh, around 2-3 minutes for each side.

5. Serve promptly with hot stew oil sauce.

Garlic Shrimps With Gritted Cauliflower

Servings: 2

Cooking Time: 15 Minutes

Ingredients:

For Preparing Shrimps

1 Pound Shrimps

2-3tbsp Cajun seasoning

Salt

1tbsp Butter/Ghee

For Preparing Cauliflower Grits

2tbsp Ghee

12-Ounces of Cauliflower

1 Garlic clove

Salt-to-taste

Directions:

1. Boil cauliflower and garlic in 8ounces of water on medium flame until it's tender.

2. Blend tender cauliflower in the food processor with ghee. Add steaming water gradually for the right consistency.

3. Sprinkle 2tbsp of Cajun seasoning on shrimps and marinate.

4. In a large skillet, take 3tbsp of ghee and cook shrimps on medium flame.

5. Place a large spoon of cauliflower grits in bowl top up with fried shrimps.

Nutrition Info: Calories 107 Carbs: 1g Fat: 3g Protein: 20g

Broccoli Tuna _Servings: 1_

Cooking Time: 10 Minutes

Ingredients:

1 tsp. Extra Virgin Olive Oil

3oz. Tuna in water, preferably light & chunky, drained 1 tbsp. Walnuts, chopped coarsely

2 cups Broccoli, chopped finely

½ tsp. Hot Sauce

Directions:

1. Begin by mixing broccoli, seasoning & tuna in a large-sized mixing bowl until they are well combined.

2. Then, microwave the veggies in the oven for 3 minutes or until tender

3. Then, stir in the walnuts and olive oil to the bowl and mix well.

4. Serve and enjoy.

Nutrition Info: Calories 259Kcal Proteins:27.1g Carbohydrates: 12.9g Fat: 12.4g

Butternut Squash Soup With Shrimp _Servings: 4_

Cooking Time: 20 Minutes

Ingredients:

3 tablespoons unsalted butter

1 small red onion, finely chopped

1 garlic clove, sliced

1 teaspoon turmeric

1 teaspoon salt

¼ teaspoon freshly ground black pepper

3 cups vegetable broth

2 cups peeled butternut squash cut into ¼-inch dice 1-pound cooked peeled shrimp, thawed if necessary 1 cup unsweetened almond milk

¼ cup slivered almonds (optional)

2 tablespoons finely chopped fresh flat-leaf parsley 2 teaspoons grated or minced lemon zest

Directions:

1. Dissolve the butter over high heat in a large pot.

2. Add the onion, garlic, turmeric, salt, and pepper and sauté until the vegetables are soft and translucent, 5 to 7 minutes.

3. Add the broth and squash and boil.

4. Simmer within 5 minutes.

5. Add the shrimp and almond milk and cook until heated through about 2 minutes.

6. Sprinkle with the almonds (if using), parsley, and lemon zest and serve.

Nutrition Info: Calories 275 Total Fat: 12g Total Carbohydrates: 12g Sugar: 3g Fiber: 2g Protein: 30g Sodium: 1665mg

Tasty Turkey Baked Balls *Servings: 6*

Cooking Time: 30 Minutes

Ingredients:

1 pound ground turkey

½-cup fresh breadcrumbs, white or whole wheat ½-cup Parmesan cheese, freshly grated

½-Tbsp. basil, freshly chopped

½-Tbsp. oregano, freshly chopped

1-pc large egg, beaten

1-Tbsp. parsley, freshly chopped

3-Tbsp.s milk or water

A dash of salt and pepper

A pinch of freshly grated nutmeg

Directions:

1. Preheat your oven to 350°F.

2. Line two baking pans with parchment paper.

3. Stir in all of the ingredients in a large mixing bowl.

4. Form 1-inch balls from the mixture and place each ball in the baking pan.

5. Put the pan in the oven.

6. Bake for 30 minutes, or until the turkey cooks through and the surfaces turn brown.

7. Turn the meatballs once halfway into the cooking.

Nutrition Info: Calories: 517 CalFat: 17.2 g Protein: 38.7 g Carbs: 52.7 gFiber: 1 g

Clear Clam Chowder _Servings: 4_

Cooking Time: 15 Minutes

Ingredients:

2 tablespoons unsalted butter

2 medium carrots, cut into ½-inch pieces

2 celery stalks, thinly sliced

1 small red onion, cut into ¼-inch dice

2 garlic cloves, sliced

2 cups vegetable broth

1 (8-ounce) bottle clam juice

1 (10-ounce) can clams

½ teaspoon dried thyme

½ teaspoon salt

¼ teaspoon freshly ground black pepper

Directions:

1. Dissolve the butter in a large pot, over high heat.

2. Add the carrots, celery, onion, and garlic and sauté until slightly softened 2 to 3 minutes.

3. Add the broth and clam juice and boil.

4. Simmer and cook until the carrots are soft, 3 to 5 minutes.

5. Stir in the clams and their juices, thyme, salt, and pepper, heat through for 2 to 3 minutes, and serve.

Nutrition Info: Calories 156 Total Fat: 7g Total Carbohydrates: 7g Sugar: 3g Fiber: 1g Protein: 14g Sodium: 981mg

Rice And Chicken Pot _Servings: 4_

Cooking Time: 25 Minutes

Ingredients:

1 lb. free-range chicken breast, boneless, skinless ¼ cup of brown rice

¾ lb. mushrooms of choice, sliced

1 leek, chopped

¼ cup almonds, chopped

1 cup of water

1 Tbsp. olive oil

1 cup green beans

½ cup apple cider vinegar

2 Tbsp. all-purpose flour

1 cup milk, low fat

¼ cup Parmesan cheese, freshly grated

¼ cup sour cream

Pinch of sea salt, add more if needed

ground black pepper, to taste

Directions:

1. Pour brown rice into a pot. Add in water. Cover and bring to a boil. Lower the heat, then simmer for 30 minutes or until rice is cooked.

2. Meanwhile, in a skillet, add the chicken breast and pour just enough water to cover—season with salt. Boil the mixture, then reduce heat and allow to simmer for 10 minutes.

3. Shred the chicken. Set aside.

4. Warm the olive oil. Cook leeks until tender. Add in mushrooms.

5. Pour apple cider vinegar into the mixture. Sauté the mixture until the vinegar has evaporated. Add in flour and milk into the skillet.

Sprinkle Parmesan cheese and add in sour cream. Season with black pepper.

6. Preheat the oven to 350 degrees F. lightly grease a casserole dish with oil.

7. Spread cooked rice in the casserole dish, then the shredded chicken and green beans on top. Add mushrooms and leeks sauce.

Put almonds on top.

8. Bake within 20 minutes or until golden brown. Allow cooling before serving.

Nutrition Info: Calories 401 Carbs: 54g Fat: 12g Protein: 20g

Sautéed Shrimp Jambalaya Jumble _Servings: 4_

Cooking Time: 30 Minutes

Ingredients:

10-oz. medium shrimp, peeled

¼-cup celery, chopped ½-cup onion, chopped

1-Tbsp. oil or butter ¼-tsp garlic, minced

¼-tsp onion salt or sea salt

⅓-cup tomato sauce ½-tsp smoked paprika

½-tsp Worcestershire sauce

⅔-cup carrots, chopped

1¼-cups chicken sausage, precooked and diced 2-cups lentils, soaked overnight and precooked 2-cups okra, chopped

A dash of crushed red pepper and black pepper Parmesan cheese, grated for topping (optional) Directions:

1. Sauté the shrimp, celery, and onion with oil in a pan placed over medium-high heat for five minutes, or until the shrimp turn pinkish.

2. Add in the rest of the ingredients, and sauté further for 10

minutes, or until the veggies are tender.

3. To serve, divide the jambalaya mixture equally among four serving bowls.

4. Top with pepper and cheese, if desired.

Nutrition Info: Calories: 529Fat: 17.6gProtein: 26.4gCarbs: 98.4gFiber: 32.3g

Chicken Chili _Servings: 6_

Cooking Time: 1 Hour

Ingredients:

1 yellow onion, chopped

2 tablespoons olive oil

2 garlic cloves, minced

1-pound chicken breast, skinless, boneless and cubed 1 green bell pepper, chopped

2 cups chicken stock

1 tablespoon cocoa powder

2 tablespoons chili powder

1 teaspoon smoked paprika

1 cup canned tomatoes, chopped

1 tablespoon cilantro, chopped

A pinch of salt and black pepper

Directions:

1. Heat up a pot with the oil over medium heat, add the onion and the garlic and sauté for 5 minutes.

2. Add the meat and brown it for 5 minutes more.

3. Add the rest of the ingredients, toss, cook over medium heat for 40 minutes.

4. Divide the chili into bowls and serve for lunch.

Nutrition Info: calories 300, fat 2, fiber 10, carbs 15, protein 11

Garlic And Lentil Soup *Servings: 4*

Cooking Time: 15 Minutes

Ingredients:

2 tablespoons extra-virgin olive oil

2 medium carrots, thinly sliced

1 small white onion, cut into ¼-inch dice

2 garlic cloves, thinly sliced

1 teaspoon ground cinnamon

1 teaspoon salt

¼ teaspoon freshly ground black pepper

3 cups vegetable broth

1 (15-ounce) can lentils, drained and rinsed 1 tablespoon minced or grated orange zest

¼ cup chopped walnuts (optional)

2 tablespoons finely chopped fresh flat-leaf parsley Directions:

1. Heat-up the oil over high heat in a large pot.

2. Put the carrots, onion, and garlic and sauté until softened, 5 to 7 minutes.

3. Put the cinnamon, salt, and pepper and stir to coat the vegetables, 1 to 2 minutes evenly.

4. Put the broth and boil. Simmer, then put the lentils, and cook until within 1 minute.

5. Stir in the orange zest and serve, sprinkled with the walnuts (if using) and parsley.

Nutrition Info: Calories 201 Total Fat: 8g Total Carbohydrates: 22g Sugar: 4g Fiber: 8g Protein: 11g Sodium: 1178mg

Zesty Zucchini & Chicken In Classic Santa Fe Stir-fry

Servings: 2

Cooking Time: 15 Minutes

Ingredients:

1-Tbsp. olive oil

2-pcs chicken breasts, sliced

1-pc onion, small, diced

2-cloves garlic, minced 1-pc zucchini, diced ½- cup carrots, shredded

1-tsp paprika, smoked 1-tsp cumin, ground

½-tsp chili powder ¼-tsp sea salt

2-Tbsp. fresh lime juice

¼-cup cilantro, freshly chopped

Brown rice or quinoa, when serving

Directions:

1. Sauté the chicken with olive oil for about 3 minutes until the chicken turns brown. Set aside.

2. Use the same wok and add the onion and garlic.

3. Cook until the onion is tender.

4. Add in the carrots and zucchini.

5. Stir the mixture, and cook further for about a minute.

6. Add all the seasonings into the mix, and stir to cook for another minute.

7. Return the chicken in the wok, and pour in the lime juice.

8. Stir to cook until everything cooks through.

9. To serve, place the mixture over cooked rice or quinoa and top with the freshly chopped cilantro.

Nutrition Info: Calories: 191Fat: 5.3gProtein: 11.9gCarbs: 26.3gFiber: 2.5g

Tilapia Tacos With Awesome Ginger-sesame Slaw

Servings: 4

Cooking Time: 5 Hours

Ingredients:

1 tsp fresh ginger, grated

Salt and freshly cracked black pepper to taste 1 tsp stevia

1 tbsp soy sauce

1 tbsp olive oil

1 tbsp lemon juice

1 tbsp plain yogurt

1½lb tilapia fillets

1 cup coleslaw mix

Directions:

1. Switch on the instant pot, add all the ingredients in it, except for tilapia fillets and coleslaw mix, and stir until well combined.

2. Then add fillets, toss until well coated, shut with the lid, press the

'slow cook' button, and cook for 5 hours, flipping the fillets halfway through.

3. When done, transfer fillets to a dish and let cool completely.

4. For meal prep, distribute coleslaw mix between four air-tight containers, add tilapia and refrigerate for up to three days.

5. When ready to eat, reheat tilapia in the microwave until hot and then serve with coleslaw.

Nutrition Info: Calories 278, Total Fat 7.4g, Total Carbs 18.6g, Protein 35.9g, Sugar 1.2g, Fiber 8.2g, Sodium 194mg

Curry Lentil Stew _Servings: 4_

Cooking Time: 15 Minutes

Ingredients:

1 tablespoon of olive oil

1 onion, chopped

2 garlic cloves, minced

1 tablespoon of organic curry seasoning

4 cups of organic low-sodium vegetable broth 1 cup of red lentils

2 cups of butternut squash, cooked

1 cup of kale

1 teaspoon of turmeric

Sea salt to taste

Directions:

1. Sauté the olive oil with the onion and garlic in a large pot over medium heat, add. Sauté for 3 minutes.

2. Add in the organic curry seasoning, vegetable broth, and lentils, and bring to a boil—Cook for 10 minutes.

3. Stir in the cooked butternut squash and kale.

4. Add in the turmeric and sea salt to taste.

5. Serve warm.

<u>Nutrition Info:</u> Total Carbohydrates 41g Dietary Fiber: 13g Protein: 16g Total Fat: 4g Calories: 252

Kale Caesar Salad With Grilled Chicken Wrap

Servings: 2

Cooking Time: 20 Minutes

Ingredients:

6 cups curly kale, cut into small, bite-sized pieces ½ coddled egg; cooked

8 ounces grilled chicken, thinly sliced

½ teaspoon Dijon mustard

¾ cup Parmesan cheese, finely shredded

ground black pepper

kosher salt

1 garlic clove, minced

1 cup cherry tomatoes, quartered

1/8 cup lemon juice, freshly squeezed

2 large tortillas or two Lavash flatbreads

1 teaspoon agave or honey

1/8 cup olive oil

Directions:

1. Combine half of the coddled egg with mustard, minced garlic, honey, olive oil, and lemon juice in a large-sized mixing bowl. Whisk until you get dressing like consistency. Season with pepper and salt to taste.

2. Add the cherry tomatoes, chicken and kale; gently toss until nicely coated with the dressing & then add ¼ cup of parmesan.

3. Spread out the flatbreads & evenly distribute the prepared salad on top of the wraps; sprinkle each with approximately ¼ cup of the parmesan.

4. Roll up the wraps & slice into half. Serve immediately & enjoy.

Nutrition Info: kcal 511 Fat: 29 g Fiber: 2.8 g Protein: 50 g

Spinach Bean Salad *Servings: 1*

Cooking Time: 5 Minutes

Ingredients:

1 cup of fresh spinach

¼ cup of canned black beans

½ cup of canned garbanzo beans

½ cup of cremini mushrooms

2 tablespoons of organic balsamic vinaigrette 1 tablespoon of olive oil

Directions:

1. Cook the cremini mushrooms with the olive oil over low, medium heat for 5 minutes, until lightly browned.

2. Assemble the salad by adding the fresh spinach to a plate and topping it with the beans, mushrooms, and the balsamic vinaigrette.

Nutrition Info: Total Carbohydrates 26gg Dietary Fiber: 8g Protein: 9g Total Fat: 15g Calories: 274

Crusted Salmon With Walnuts & Rosemary

Servings: 6

Cooking Time: 20 Minutes

Ingredients:

1 Mince garlic clove

1tbsp Dijon mustard

¼ tbsp Lemon zest

1tbsp Lemon juice

1tbsp fresh rosemary

1/2 tbsp Honey

Olive oil

Fresh parsley

3tbsp Chopped walnuts

1 Pound skinless salmon

1tbsp Fresh crushed red pepper

Salt & pepper

Lemon wedges for garnish

3tbsp Panko breadcrumbs

1tbsp extra-virgin olive oil

Directions:

1. Spread the baking sheet in the oven and preheat it at 240C.

2. In a bowl, mix mustard paste, garlic, salt, olive oil, honey, lemon juice, crushed red pepper, rosemary, pus honey.

3. Combine panko, walnuts, and oil and spread thin fish slice on the baking sheet. Spray olive oil equally on both sides of the fish.

4. Place walnut mixture on the salmon with the mustard mixture on top it.

5. Bake the salmon almost for 12 minutes. Garnish it with fresh parsley and lemon wedges and serve it hot.

Nutrition Info: Calories 227 Carbs: 0g Fat: 12g Protein: 29g

Baked Sweet Potato With Red Tahini Sauce

Servings: 4

Cooking Time: 30 Minutes

Ingredients:

15-ounces Canned Chickpeas

4 Medium-sized sweet potatoes

½ tbsp Olive oil

1 Pinch salt

1tbsp Lime juice

1/2 tbsp of cumin, coriander, and paprika powder For Garlic Herb Sauce

¼ Cup tahini sauce

½ tbsp Lime Juice

3 cloves garlic

Salt to taste

Directions:

1. Preheat the oven at 204°C. Toss chickpeas in salt, spices & olive oil. Spread them on the foil sheet.

2. Brush sweet potato thin wedges with oil and place them on marinated beans and bake.

3. For the sauce, mix all fixings in a bowl. Add some water in it, but keep it thick.

4. Remove sweet potatoes from the oven after 25 minutes.

5. Garnish this baked sweet potato chickpea salad with hot garlic sauce.

Nutrition Info: Calories 90 Carbs: 20g Fat: 0g Protein: 2g

Italian Summer Squash Soup *Servings: 4*

Cooking Time: 15 Minutes

Ingredients:

3 tablespoons extra-virgin olive oil

1 small red onion, thinly sliced

1 garlic clove, minced

1 cup shredded zucchini

1 cup shredded yellow squash

½ cup shredded carrot

3 cups vegetable broth

1 teaspoon salt

2 tablespoons finely chopped fresh basil

1 tablespoon finely chopped fresh chives

2 tablespoons pine nuts

Directions:

1. Heat-up the oil over high heat in a large pot.

2. Put the onion and garlic and sauté until softened, 5 to 7 minutes.

3. Add the zucchini, yellow squash, and carrot and sauté until softened, 1 to 2 minutes.

4. Add the broth and salt, and boil. Simmer within 1 to 2 minutes.

5. Stir in the basil and chives and serve, sprinkled with the pine nuts.

Nutrition Info: Calories 172 Total Fat: 15g Total Carbohydrates: 6g Sugar: 3g Fiber: 2g Protein: 5g Sodium: 1170mg

Saffron And Salmon Soup Servings: 4

Cooking Time: 20 Minutes

Ingredients:

¼ cup extra-virgin olive oil

2 leeks, white parts only, thinly sliced

2 medium carrots, thinly sliced

2 garlic cloves, thinly sliced

4 cups vegetable broth

1-pound skinless salmon fillets, cut into 1-inch pieces 1 teaspoon salt

¼ teaspoon freshly ground black pepper

¼ teaspoon saffron threads

2 cups baby spinach

½ cup dry white wine

2 tablespoons chopped scallions, both white and green parts 2 tablespoons finely chopped fresh flat-leaf parsley Directions:

1. Heat the oil over high in a large pot.

2. Add the leeks, carrots, and garlic and sauté until softened, 5 to 7 minutes.

3. Put the broth and boil.

4. Simmer and add the salmon, salt, pepper, and saffron. Cook until the salmon is cooked through, about 8 minutes.

5. Add the spinach, wine, scallions, and parsley and cook until the spinach has wilted, 1 to 2 minutes, and serve.

Nutrition Info: Calories 418 Total Fat: 26g Total Carbohydrates: 13g Sugar: 4g Fiber: 2g Protein: 29g Sodium: 1455mg

Thai Flavored Hot And Sour Shrimp And Mushroom Soup

Servings: 6

Cooking Time: 38 Minutes

Ingredients:

3 tbsp unsalted butter

1lb shrimp, peeled and deveined

2 tsp minced garlic

1-inch piece ginger root, peeled

1 medium onion, diced

1 red Thai chili, chopped

1 lemongrass stalk

½ tsp fresh lime zest

Salt and freshly cracked black pepper, to taste 5 cups chicken broth

1 tbsp coconut oil

½lb cremini mushrooms, sliced into wedges

1 small green zucchini

2 tbsp fresh lime juice

2 tbsp fish sauce

¼ bunch of fresh Thai basil, chopped

¼ bunch of fresh cilantro, chopped

Directions:

1. Take a large pot, place it over medium heat, add butter and when it melts, add shrimps, garlic, ginger, onion, chilies, lemongrass, and lime zest, season with salt and black pepper and cook for 3 minutes.

2. Pour in broth, simmer for 30 minutes, and then strain it.

3. Take a large skillet pan over medium heat, add oil and when hot, add mushrooms and zucchini, season more with salt and black pepper and cook for 3 minutes.

4. Add shrimp's mixture in the skillet pan, simmer for 2 minutes, drizzle with lime juice and fish sauce and cook for 1 minute.

5. Taste to adjust seasoning, then remove the pan from heat, garnish with cilantro and basil and serve.

Nutrition Info: Calories 223, Total Fat 10.2g, Total Carbs 8.7g, Protein 23g, Sugar 3.6g, Sodium 1128mg

Orzo With Sundried Tomatoes Ingredients:

1 lb boneless skinless chicken bosoms, diced into 3/4-inch pieces

1 Tbsp + 1 tsp olive oil

Salt and crisply ground dark pepper

2 cloves garlic, minced

1/4 cups (8 oz) dry orzo pasta

2 3/4 cups low-sodium chicken stock, at that point more varying (don't utilize ordinary juices, it will be excessively salty) 1/3 cup sun dried tomato parts stuffed in oil with herbs (around 12 parts. Shake off a portion of the abundance oil), hacked fine in a nourishment processor

1/2 - 3/4 cup finely destroyed parmesan cheddar, to taste 1/3 cup cleaved crisp basil

Directions:

1. Warmth 1 Tbsp olive oil in a saute container over medium-high warmth.

2. Once gleaming include chicken, season gently with salt and pepper and cook until brilliant, around 3 minutes at that point pivot to inverse sides and cook until brilliant dark colored and cooked through, around 3 minutes. Move chicken to a plate, spread with foil to keep warm.

3. Include staying 1 tsp olive oil to saute dish at that point include garlic and saute 20 seconds, or just until daintily brilliant, at that point pour in chicken juices while scraping up cooked bits from base of skillet.

4. Heat stock to the point of boiling at that point include orzo pasta, lessen warmth to medium spread skillet with cover and permit to delicately bubble 5 minutes at that point reveal, mix and keep on bubbling revealed until orzo is delicate, around 5 minutes longer, blending at times (don't stress if there's still a little juices, it will give it some saucy-ness).

5. When pasta has cooked through hurl chicken in with orzo at that point expel from heat. Include parmesan cheddar and mix until dissolved, at that point hurl in sun dried tomatoes, basil and season

with pepper (you shouldn't require any salt however include a little in the event that you'd think it needs it).

6. Add more juices to thin whenever wanted (as the pasta rests it will absorb abundance fluid and I enjoyed it with somewhat overabundance so I included somewhat more). Serve warm.

Mushroom And Beet Soup _Servings: 4_

Cooking Time: 40 Minutes

Ingredients:

2 tablespoons olive oil

1 yellow onion, chopped

2 beets, peeled and cut into large cubes

1-pound white mushrooms, sliced

2 garlic cloves, minced

1 tablespoon tomato paste

5 cups veggie stock

1 tablespoons parsley, chopped

Directions:

1. Heat up a pot with the oil over medium heat, add the onion and the garlic and sauté for 5 minutes.

2. Add the mushrooms, stir and sauté for 5 minutes more.

3. Add the beets and the other ingredients, bring to a simmer and cook over medium heat for 30 minutes more, stirring from time to time.

4. Ladle the soup into bowls and serve.

Nutrition Info: calories 300, fat 5, fiber 9, carbs 8, protein 7

Chicken Parmesan Meatballs_Ingredients:

2 pounds ground chicken

3/4 cup panko breadcrumbs gluten free panko will work fine 1/4 cup finely minced onion

2 tablespoons minced parsley

2 cloves garlic minced

get-up-and-go of 1 little lemon around 1 teaspoon 2 eggs

3/4 cup destroyed Pecorino Romano or Parmesan cheddar 1 teaspoon genuine salt

1/2 teaspoon crisply ground dark pepper

1 quart Five Minute Marinara Sauce

4-6 ounces mozzarella crisply cut

Directions:

1. Preheat the stove to 400 degrees, setting the rack in the upper third of the broiler. In a huge bowl, join everything aside from the marinara and the mozzarella. Softly combine, utilizing your hands or an enormous spoon. Scoop and shape into little meatballs and spot on a foil lined heating sheet. Spot the meatballs genuinely near one another on the plate to make them

fit. Spoon about a half tablespoon of sauce over every meatball. Heat for 15 minutes.

2. Expel meatballs from the stove and increment the broiler temperature to cook. Spoon an extra half tablespoon of sauce over every meatball and top with a little square of mozzarella. (I cut the slight cuts into pieces around 1" square.) Broil an extra 3 minutes, until the cheddar has softened and turned brilliant. Present with extra sauce. Appreciate!

Meatballs Alla Parmigiana_Ingredients:

For the meatballs

1.5lbs ground hamburger (80/20)

2 Tbl crisp parsley, cleaved

3/4 cup ground parmesan cheddar

1/2 cup almond flour

2 eggs

1 tsp fit salt

1/4 tsp ground dark pepper

1/4 tsp garlic powder

1 tsp dried onion drops

1/4 tsp dried oregano

1/2 cup warm water

For the Parmigiana

1 cup simple keto marinara sauce (or any sugar free locally acquired marinara)

4 oz mozzarella cheddar

Directions:

1. Join the entirety of the meatball fixings in a huge bowl and blend well.

2. Structure into fifteen 2" meatballs.

3. Prepare at 350 degrees (F) for 20 minutes OR fry in an enormous skillet over medium warmth until cooked through. Ace tip – have a go at searing in bacon oil in the event that you have any – it includes another degree of flavor. Fricasseeing produces the brilliant dark colored shading appeared in the photographs above.

4. For the Parmigiana:

5. Spot the cooked meatballs in a stove safe dish.

6. Spoon roughly 1 Tbl sauce over every meatball.

7. Spread with roughly 1/4 oz of mozzarella cheddar each.

8. Prepare at 350 degrees (F) for 20 minutes (40 minutes if meatballs are solidified) or until warmed through and the cheddar is brilliant.

9. Embellishment with new parsley whenever wanted.

Sheet Pan Turkey Breast With Golden Vegetables

Servings: 4

Cooking Time: 45 Minutes

Ingredients:

2 tablespoons unsalted butter, at room temperature 1 medium acorn squash, seeded and thinly sliced 2 large golden beets, peeled and thinly sliced ½ medium yellow onion, thinly sliced

½ boneless, skin-on turkey breast (1 to 2 pounds) 2 tablespoons honey

1 teaspoon salt

1 teaspoon turmeric

¼ teaspoon freshly ground black pepper

1 cup chicken broth or vegetable broth

Directions:

1. Preheat the oven to 400°F. Grease the baking sheet with the butter.

2. Arrange the squash, beets, and onion in a single layer on the baking sheet. Put the turkey skin-side up. Drizzle with the honey.

213

Season with the salt, turmeric, and pepper, and add the broth.

3. Roast until the turkey registers 165°F in the center with an instant-read thermometer, 35 to 45 minutes. Remove, and let rest for 5 minutes.

4. Slice, and serve.

Nutrition Info: Calories 383 Total Fat: 15g Total Carbohydrates: 25g Sugar: 13g Fiber: 3g Protein: 37g Sodium: 748mg

Coconut Green Curry With Boil Rice _Servings: 8_

Cooking Time: 20 Minutes

Ingredients:

2tbsp Olive oil

12ounces of Tofu

2 medium sweet potatoes (cut into cubes)

Salt-to-taste

314ounces Coconut milk

4tbsp Green curry paste

3 Cups of Broccoli Florets

Directions:

1. Remove excess water from tofu and fry it on medium flame. Add salt in it and fry it for 12 minutes.

2. Cook coconut milk, green curry paste, and sweet potato on medium heat and simmer it for 5 mins.

3. Now add broccoli and tofu in it and cook it almost 5 minutes until the broccoli color changes.

4. Serve this coconut and green curry with a handful of boil rice and many raisins on top of it.

Nutrition Info: Calories 170 Carbs: 34g Fat: 2g Protein: 3g

Sweet Potato & Chicken Soup With Lentil

Servings: 6

Cooking Time: 35 Minutes

Ingredients:

10 Celery stalks

1 Home-cooked or rotisserie chicken

2 medium sweet potatoes

5-ounces French lentils

2tbsp Fresh lime juice

½ head bite-size escarole

6 thin-sliced garlic cloves

½ Cup dill (finely chop)

1tbsp Kosher Salt

2tbsp Extra virgin oil

Directions:

1. Add salt, chicken carcass, lentil, and sweet potatoes in 8 ounces of water and boil it on high flame.

2. Cook these items almost for 10-12 minutes and skim off all the foam form on it.

3. Cook garlic and celery in oil almost for 10 minutes until it is tender

& light brown, then add shredded roast chicken in it.

4. Add this mixture in the escarole soup and continuously stir it for 5

minutes on medium heat.

5. Add lemon juice and stir in dill. Serve season hot soup with salt.

Nutrition Info: Calories 310 Carbs: 45g Fat: 11g Protein: 13g